THE GREYSKULL LP
Second Edition

By John Sheaffer aka Johnny Pain

ISBN: 0615635571

ISBN 13: 978-0615635576

Table of Contents

Introduction

It's been over a year since I wrote 'The Greyskull LP'. The sales and distribution of the book were staggering to say the least. I honestly had no idea how far reaching the fifty-seven-page eBook would prove to be. The number of forum members on StrengthVillain.com that are applying the principles outlined in that book, and online has grown tremendously and continues to climb with each passing day.

The success stories and testimonials from those who have used the Greyskull LP come in daily via email, forum posts, and personal notes on Twitter.

Quite simply, people love the Greyskull LP.

The reasons for this are multi-pronged. For one, the method works very well in terms of building strength and muscle.

Second, the program is a set of principles, not some set-in-stone "master program" that is more effective than anything else on the planet and promises results only if you blindly adhere to its guidelines no matter how inapplicable they may actually be to you as an individual.

The flexibility of the principles allows one to design a "program" based on their desired outcomes, and what activities they enjoy.

A person seeking to lose body fat while building muscle is not laughed at and told that their outcome is impossible.

Why would we say that? We do it here all the time.

The StrengthVillain.com forum is populated by an ever-growing group of individuals who are blowing holes in many of the common myths that exist regarding what is possible in terms of strength and conditioning training. There you will find hordes of individuals who have successfully changed their bodies for the better in a variety of different ways. If you are not currently a member contributing to the forum, I highly encourage you to become one.

Flexibility is everything in training. Not in the physical sense, but in terms of changing the methods used in order to make progress in an on-going manner. Rigid programs and closed-minded coaches and individuals are not able to be flexible, and therefore come up short where we succeed.

Making progress is everything.

The Greyskull LP, the name given to the vast collection of principles and ideas used by myself to train many of my clients, some of which are presented in this book, is predicated on the idea that progress is number one.

Ego is not.

Ego will get you nowhere if you allow it to serve as your navigator.

There is information in this book that I have borrowed and stolen from others over the years. I am proud of that. I don't claim to be a strength-training visionary that has broken through long-existing barriers of knowledge on the subject and developed some earth-shattering new material.

What I have done is work hard to destroy limiting beliefs and ideas that run rampant in this industry and prevent people from getting the results that they want from their efforts.

The information presented in this book represents much of what that has manifested itself as in the physical realm. I frequently mention that the mechanics of training and diet are responsible for twenty percent of the total picture.

The other eighty percent is the mental component.

In my coaching and consulting, and in upcoming products such as "Blueprint to Beast" I teach the principles necessary to understand in order to use the eighty percent as well as any top-performer.

What you get here is the twenty-percent presented in the clearest and most concise manner that I am capable.

The principles and ideas presented here will serve as the toolbox from which you can draw knowledge and build something truly epic.

As I've stated numerous times before, make progress, the only thing we're interested in maintaining are erections.

Welcome to 'The Greyskull LP Second Edition'.

Chapter One:
Origins of the Greyskull LP

Part One

I suspect that the concept of linear progression, in relation to strength training, has existed since the dawn of time. The idea can be found in the story of the Greek wrestler Milo of Croton. Milo was said to have started hoisting a young calf to his shoulders at a young age, a practice which he continued as the calf grew to maturity, culminating in his ability to shoulder a full grown bull in his prime. Unfortunately there are no YouTube videos to substantiate those claims, but we'll take the ancient Greeks' word for it.

The point is, the concept of linear progression; adding a small amount of weight to the bar or object being lifted each time one is exposed to the stimulus, is certainly nothing new and has certainly proven its value in strength development for a very long time.

Many different incarnations of the traditional linear progression model have been presented by various sources over the years, and they all have something in common with each other besides the obvious addition of weight to the bar in small increments. That is they work…

…at least for a while.

So if it's understood that linear progression is gold for a beginner lifter, and that it is accepted by everyone that the concept will not work indefinitely (lest everyone be 10,000 lb squatters in a few years of training) why go tampering with the idea? If it aint broke don't fix it right? Just accept that you should squeeze as much out of the traditional linear progression concept before needing to use more sophisticated and complex methods to continue to make progress in strength or muscle growth.

That's the part I always had a problem with.

Why do we abandon the most basic premise in training after a few weeks or months and simply 'accept' that our ability to drive progress with a simple method, predicated on the idea that we need to be doing something we haven't done before every time we step in the gym, has ended, and that we must seek out a more complicated method with a cooler name? Simple, because someone says so, that's why.

It's never been in my nature to do much of anything because someone said so, and so to the drawing board I went.

Let's look at the popular three sets of five across model, used by many these days. The lifter performs the given lifts for the prescribed three sets of five reps in a series of workouts throughout the week, adding a set amount of weight to the bar with each successive workout, until the ability to do so ceases and the trainee 'hits a wall'. This is the very approach that I myself used in gaining a significant amount of size and strength when I committed to doing so. I was a devout follower, and did not deviate from the program. I can honestly say that those months were some of the most productive training months I have ever experienced, and like all decisions that I have learned and grown from, I certainly do not regret having trained in that manner.

What did predictably happen, as I expected it would, is that I eventually reached a point where I was unable to continue making the progress described above.. This was normal and to be accepted. I did everything I could to prolong the inevitable and shift to more complicated, less rewarding training. I was advised by conventional wisdom to take a shot at a few 'resets', periods of time in which the bar weight was reduced by a percentage and some of the cumulative fatigue brought on by the previous weeks of stout workload was allowed to subside while performing some 'easy' or 'light' workouts.

This was the first part I had significant issue with.

The invigorating, 'let me at the weights' attitude I had for the many prior training weeks was gone. The fire to get in the gym, get under the bar and smash into new territory wasn't there. Instead I was left with a compulsion to go the gym and go through the motions of a weight training session, knowing I had already conquered these weights and that if I followed the schedule it would be several weeks of sessions before I broke into new territory again. The Viking in me was greatly displeased and discouraged with the prospect of this, although I plugged along according to plan, only to find myself back at the same wall I had encountered a few weeks prior. I passed the point at which I had stuck, but only by a few pounds, and the thought of enduring another reset seemed less pleasant than a root canal (an association that is ingrained in many and one that I daily work to break in others through my consulting business). This was very disheartening and did not do much for my motivation to try the same method again, seeing as how my face was still sore from backing up a few steps, before running into the wall this time.

So what was I to do? Well, I did what I was supposed to and moved on to more 'advanced' programming. Here I found myself participating in workouts lasting well over an hour and left me beat up and genuinely disinterested in training. My killer instinct to progress with the barbell was gone. I lacked the both the intrinsic and extrinsic (bar weight) rewards I had been receiving from training previously. I was, perhaps predictably, not performing well at all during my sessions. I found myself missing workouts for the first time in months with increasing consistency. Then the inevitable happened.

I quit.

Yep, gave it up. Well, just for a week or so, and only the traditional linear progression method. I returned to the gym armed with a 'program' inspired by Dorian Yates, among others. I began doing exercises I hadn't done in months because they weren't part of 'the program'. I started experimenting with different rep ranges and different spins on the movements and guess what? I loved it.

I was having fun again. The fire was back; records were falling, as was the time spent in the gym, seeing as how I was not waiting around getting ready for the attempt to grind out yet another heavy set of five reps on my lifts, beat myself up day after day. Not only was I gaining muscle again, but my waist measurement was shrinking. I had altered my diet, tightening it up from the method of caloric surplus that was traditionally advocated as an accompaniment to the program(s) I had been performing. I went back to what I knew diet wise, and what kept me amped about training in the program department. I firmly believe that even the best program in the world is useless to a trainee the minute they find it boring. Over the next year and beyond I continued doing what I wanted to do, drawing on my experience and knowledge from years of an obsession with strength training and the results just kept coming. Having had a background in bodybuilding, I saw serious holes in my physique that had developed as result of neglecting certain exercises for so long. I filled those gaps nicely with the use of traditional tools and exercises that others condemned or deemed silly. Hey, I didn't care, I was pushing 240 at 5'11" and my 40" waist was down to 37.5" with my lifts still climbing (past the 200/300/400/500 standards that are recognized by many).

All was well in the world of Johnny Pain.

In my business, I was still applying to others the method that I had used to gain and to grow. I kept prescribing the same 3 x 5 basic template to trainees and was predictably getting good results. I was also eventually getting into the same troubles as I had encountered: people were getting jammed up, hurt and losing the necessary motivation and momentum to progress within an increasingly predictable amount of time. This was accepted as normal and since I had experienced the same I tried to 'fix' the mistakes I had made in my own training, in the programming of others. This proved to be both detrimental (temporarily) to some in terms of their progress (I'm also not too proud to say that I lost a few clients out of sheer boredom with their training and progress) and incredibly valuable in terms of the experience and virtual laboratory that I had at my disposal.

I smartened up quickly (I'm good like that) and realized that I was not this special flower who was just different than everyone else in how my mind and body responded to what was asked of it. I realized that others were suffering from the same bored, borderline overtrained, beat down condition that I myself had fallen into. From a conditioning perspective they weren't terribly impressive either. Most would get disheartened while attempting something that challenged them cardiovascularly because they felt they had regressed in condition from before they went on their quest (under my lead) for newfound strength. I knew that it was selfish and unfair of me to allow myself the pleasure of actually enjoying my training and getting the results I wanted, while my clients who I genuinely cared about, and who respected, looked up to, trusted, and PAID me languished in this limbo of unproductive boredom after their initial fling with progress was over.

Some things had to change.

I took a good look at what was fundamentally effective from the programs I was using prior to this 'awakening'. The focus on the basic barbell lifts was a critical component, as was the concept of simple linear progression. The simplistic design could be tweaked a lot I thought, however, and the fear of overtraining that was instilled in all of us could be quelled. Conditioning sessions could be added and would not have to be taboo. Recovery would not be affected drastically if the advocated diets were better and if the additional work was 'layered in' (a concept I have always embraced and use with every single one of my trainees in one capacity or another). Squats need not be performed every session in order to make progress, in fact I found the opposite to be true, more significant results were hade and over a longer training period when one squatting session was eliminated completely. Accessory or 'beach work' was added to fill the physique gaps before they developed (let's face it, even the most *form follows function* indoctrinated individuals want to look good, aesthetically, on some level). The big lift of the day could be done last (as I had always done in bodybuilding workouts) so as to let you cry on the floor for a few minutes upon completion, rather than saddle up and attempt to muster the energy necessary to go on and train a smaller muscle group (which chronically and visibly lagged behind in development in proponents of the previously used methods). All of these changes were proving to be money. Everyone was happy, as was I. Progress was great, focus was back, energy and mood were at an all time high.

But there was still one problem. Everyone would still get stuck at some point.

Enter 'The Greyskull Reset'

I had long been a fan of intensity-based training (I already paid homage to Dorian once in this book) and its proponents. I liked the idea of giving it my all, leaving nothing in the tank. I guess it is just part of my personality, but I have always been able to get fired up to do just a little bit better than before if it was at all physically possible. I've observed that most are like that as well. Maybe not at first, but we can always get it out of them.

The problem I had, which I mentioned before, with the conventional method of resetting was that so much time was spent treading over territory that had already been conquered. There were huge gaps between productive workouts (on paper at least). I found that others and myself had dreaded resetting, and therefore avoided them like the plague, often risking injury by attempting to add too much weight and perform movements in a less than safe manner in the name of continued progression and avoiding a reset.

I began to have my people rep out the last of their three sets during their resets (when they had taken 10% off of the weight that they could not successfully complete for three sets of five). This was a critical factor.. The energy was great, they were training with a ton of intensity and busting their balls (ovaries if they were women, everybody's got gonads) to set a new rep record, or tie the number of reps they got the workout before, except with more weight this time. The sticking points were falling by significant margins. Tested maxes (for data collection) of 'stuck' individuals were improving dramatically after returning to the weight that had humbled them before the reset.

The case of one trainee in particular is illuminating. He had been unable to get three sets of five at 300 in the squat previously. After taking 10% off the bar the trainee got 270 for nine on his first workout. He was able to hold the rep max set at nine for several workouts despite adding five pounds to the bar each time. I then tested him a few days later for a one rep amx: 340 was the magic number. He smashed 300 for seven when he got back to it, and later still tested a one rep max of 365! Yes, a 25 lb increase without ever adding more weight to the bar.

Maximal strength was increasing during the resets, no longer were we just spinning our wheels for a few weeks taking easy workouts waiting for the shot to get back in the game. We were seeing people get stronger while using less weight on the bar. The best part? Their motivation was crazy. The rep maxes were a challenge. It wasn't a 'reset' anymore; it was a fun 'rep max phase'.

At the time I would have the trainee return to three sets of five once they had broken new ground. This was mainly political due to associations I had at the time with an organization headed by an individual whom had been one of the foremost proponents of that method. I began to question why I would have someone who was capable of seven reps with a given weight artificially terminate the set at five, a seemingly arbitrary number. It didn't make much sense to me.

At the same time another significant revelation came about. I had been noticing that some clients were experiencing very good hypertrophy during these resets. Several of my consult clients who had used this method early on were noticing the same. They were very happy with the growth that they were seeing during these periods of their training. Then one day, while having an impromptu 'posedown' in the mirror at Greyskull, one of my young high school kids (a tenth grader at the time) said to me "I need to get some more size on my upper body", (he was making the remark comparing his upper body development to mine) he continued: "Do you think I could do another reset?"

That sentence sealed the deal for me. Here was a kid whose only exposure to lifting had come from me, and from his high school football team's program, which was let's just say less than stellar, and he was expressing to me his desire to reset his lifts again.

In order to grow.

He was associating the 'resets' with growth. It wasn't just me, I wasn't crazy, these kids were seeing through crystal clear, unbiased, glass that they were growing and getting stronger during their resets than they were during their 'three sets of five' training periods.

Then the revelation that had been sitting dormant in my mind, that I had pushed aside because I knew it was blasphemous, elbowed its way to the forefront of my consciousness,

"Why not just train them like they're resetting all the time?"

This was the tipping point. This question was the drug that induced labor.

Johnny Pain gave birth, naturally, to what would later be dubbed the "Greyskull LP" on the dirty concrete floor of Greyskull Barbell Club minutes later.

Part Two

Many very satisfied clients later the Greyskull LP method began to gain further momentum over the internet, in an unexpected manner.

I was the 'Nutrition Guy' on a popular website, I had a Q and A section as a 'Guest Coach' and would answer all questions pertaining to diet for the forum's members. Occasionally I would get a training question thrown in here and there (the training questions generally went to the site's host) but it was mostly related to my dietary expertise. Interestingly enough the dietary recommendations I would make on that site were often a lot tighter than I make on my site StrengthVillain.com or with my consult clients. Why you ask? Because the accepted practice over there was that one would weight train using the methods prescribed by the site's owner and do little else, lest they sacrifice strength gains or overtrain. Seeing as how most additional activities were considered taboo or at the very least not conducive, if not detrimental, to progress much of the dietary 'wiggle room' afforded to the hard training athlete who lifted weights and competed in sports, or at least performed some sort of conditioning work a few times per week, was not present. Many were in danger of becoming a sloppy mess. Adhering to a tight, bodybuilder-style, diet was the best way that I could help these guys and gals not pack on excessive fat with the muscle, as well as strip the fat off if it was too late.

It was clear that some of the training recommendations I'd often make in response to the more direct questions about my methods upset the status quo in that house. This was not a large-scale problem by any means, as I mentioned before, few asked for my advice on training anyway. It was significant enough however for some to take notice of the inconsistencies in the ideas, and ask for more bits and pieces of the big picture methods we used here in my gym. Little by little some of the ideas I had found to work well got discussed and I began to receive a few more training enquiries in the forum.

At the same time, the volume of consulting I was doing increased quite a bit, largely due to my presence on said forum. Most would contact me, 'happy' with their training methods and programs, but unhappy with the accumulated fat and the stalled progress. In the beginning it was a host of individuals who did not want to hear my blasphemous ideas on why they were stuck or how to break the walls down, but eventually the demographic of individuals calling me became an information thirsty bunch willing to give a new idea a shot that they felt sounded logical. I started applying my 'Greyskull Resets' to all of the people who contacted me. I was batting a thousand in the department of getting people unstuck.

Wednesday squat sessions were dropped, and all lifts were reset. This took place within the first few minutes of the call. Dietary guidance was of course given, and provided much value in terms of getting everything to work together nicely, but the overwhelming majority of feedback from my clients was how much fun they were having in their sessions and how happy they were to be making progress again.

A thread was started by Dan Miguelez, a great guy and long time supporter of mine as a place for people to park their testimonials from their consult experiences. The posts came in with regularity, unsolicited following the consults, and all were from satisfied customers. They were making gains, losing fat, smashing PRs, and most importantly having fun while they were doing it. It was rapidly becoming clear to the other board members by this point that I had a lot of expertise and knowledge to contribute on the training, as well as, the diet front.

Then one day an older guy (late 40s, early 50s I believe) asked me about pre, during, and post-workout nutrition for older trainees. He said his sessions were now taking him close to two hours and that he found his energy was tapering halfway through his workout (big surprise!). He wanted a dietary fix for this, something he could drink that would boost his energy and allow him to trudge back through the second half of his lengthy, high volume, day. I battled with whether or not to tell him that I thought the problem was with his program and not his diet, since he was training in the proprietary the way of the shop owner over there. Eventually, honesty won out. I told him my thoughts. He asked me how I would go about amending his program to better suit his individual needs and I jotted down some of my recommendations in a forum post.

That thread gained momentum in a big hurry. Days later the thread was still active and gaining posts. For three weeks I did not get a single diet related question, everyone wanted to know more about the methods I was using and how they could apply them to get the results others were enjoying. Other sites started to link to that thread, and discussion boards were chatting about it as well. There was definitely a buzz about the whole thing.

Enter StrengthVillain.com

Fast-forward a few weeks. The owner of the website and I agreed to go our separate ways and I had decided that I needed a place to host my Q and A. It was a big source of exposure for me and honestly drove a lot of my income at the time through the consultations that would come from readers wanting me to custom tailor their diet and program (a practice I still enjoy and engage in with regularity). StrengthVillain.com was born and with it a new forum which now featured a Q and A section with not only myself, but also Jim Wendler, and University of Penn Strength Coach Jim Steel. I was proud of my new baby and worked around the clock to build it up. Many of the people who had followed my stuff on the other site now populated my board. Many who kept training logs over there packed up shop and relocated their logs to StrengthVillain. As expected with a site that delivers quality content, membership increased rapidly and a new, thriving, forum was present in the midst of the other big strength training forums.

Here I was free to say and do what I wanted. The gloves came off and I answered every question, even those about controversial or illegal subjects with 100% honesty. There were no shortage of training questions over here, and no shortage of information being communicated from my end. The Greyskull Methods were out in the open now, on a much larger scale, and the people were very satisfied. For many it was great to hear that they weren't abnormal for wanting a nice pair of arms, or for wanting a waistline that they could be proud of. People weren't berated or put down for expressing desire to be able to do more than lift weights, or to compete in a 5k race with coworkers. It was a new home for many and a haven for like-minded individuals.

It was in my Q and A section that the term 'Greyskull LP' started to be used. At first I disliked the name, but like Dante Trudel whose moniker 'DoggCrapp' has stuck since his first post (which was to be his only) on a bodybuilding forum turned into a huge, several hundred-page thread, I grew to accept it and embrace it. One day a poster asked for a concise explanation of "the program", something I had avoided doing for a while since there were individual differences in the layout based on the person's goals. I am not one to disappoint however, and although it was late and I was running on fumes, I obliged him and scribbled down a version of the method that I thought was as generally applicable to my readers as possible. As it stands today (March 2, 2011) that thread, which has since been stickied and which was started on November 2, 2010, has over 450 replies, is over 46 pages in length, and has been viewed close to 30,000 times (at press time on this, the second edition, the thread has over 1,400 replies, is 141 pages in length, and has been viewed close to 132,000 times). Not unlike Dante's 'Cycles on Pennies' thread, the Greyskull LP thread gained some serious steam and has helped a significant amount of people.

After telling everyone to wait for 'By The Power!', my big encyclopedia of the Greyskull Methods, to come out later in the year and shed some light on the program (2ed note: 'By the Power' has yet to be released), as well as many others, people still asked me regularly to put out an eBook on the topic of the Greyskull LP*. Never one to let down my supporters, here we are.[1]

---

[1] For the record you can thank a short (though very strong), smart assed Recon Marine at one of my seminars who was insanely jealous of my fly- ass sneakers for being the proverbial straw that broke the camel's back. His was the request for an in-my-own-words, clear, concise write up of the intricacies of this program that made me decide once and for all to release this.

Chapter Two:
"What is the Greyskull LP?"

Ok, so if we're going to put a name on this thing, let's define what it is that we're talking about when we do so…

What is the 'Greyskull LP'?

Let's talk about some of the principle characteristics of the base program, and then in the later chapters we will get into the add-ons. I like to use a software analogy here: the base set of ideas being the fundamental 'software program', and the other layers being 'plug ins' that can be added or removed based on the individual needs of the trainee.
So let's have a look at the principle characteristics of the base program.

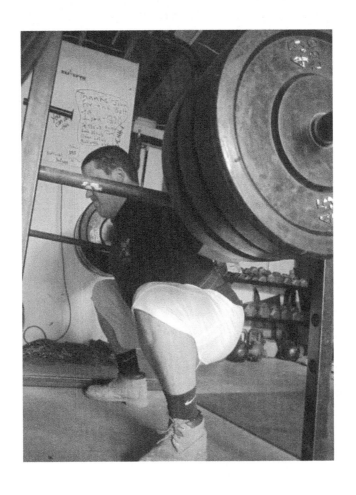

Section One: Exposure Frequency by Lift

We'll begin by looking at the frequency with which the lifts are performed in the conventional version.

-The squat is performed on the first and third days of the base, three day per week, program.

-The deadlift is performed on the second (middle) training day of the week.

-The press and the bench press (or their substitutes) are executed in an alternating (A/B) fashion each training day. For instance, on the first week, (assuming a Monday, Wednesday, Friday layout) the bench press may be executed on Monday and again on Friday, while the press would be done on Wednesday. The following week, the pressing sessions would take place in the Monday and Friday workouts, while the bench press would take place once that week, on Wednesday.

"But JP, why not squat three times per week?"

As I mentioned in the origins chapter, one of the intentions of this program is to provide what I call 'longevity of progress'. I am a firm believer in making sure training progression is appropriately paced to ensure consistent strength gains over a long period of time, as well as optimizing recovery which directly influences long term progression.

Someone endeavoring to squat three times per week, while adding 10 lbs to the bar each workout, is adding 30 lbs per week to their training weight. No one pretends that this pace can be maintained for a long period of time – I realize but if we do extrapolate those figures, we see that a 30 lb increase in training weight over the course of six months would result in 720 lbs added to the initial training poundage! Clearly even the weakest of beginners with the highest ambitions and the sloppiest gross caloric intakes will be unable to maintain that pace for long. If they were we'd all be walking around with 800-pound-plus squats

If we reduce that number to five pounds per session, and squat three times per week, this brings the six-month projected increase in training weight down to 360 lbs. Still out of reach as a realistic linear increase for sure.

Now let's take that a step further and add five pounds to the bar twice per week for a total of 10 lbs added to the bar weekly. What does that yield us in 6 months? 240 lbs. Are we getting realistic yet?

Yes and No.

Taking a squat from 135 for five to 375 for five could potentially be accomplished in six months, and I'm sure it has been done. However the likelihood of that happening in my experience is slim, assuming that 135 represents a stimulus for the trainee and they are lifting without the aid of anabolics. So then a series of questions needs to be asked in order to bring all of this together and have it make sense.

Q: Does it matter if we keep the pace and make all 240 lbs of progress in bar weight in the six-month period?

A: *No it doesn't.*

Q: *Do we set out to do that?*

A: *No we don't.*

So if we know that we are not going to be able to keep the pace anyway, why don't we step on it a bit and increase the jumps between sessions so that we at least get to a heavier bar weight sooner?

The simple answer is because we are not using bar weight as the only variable to drive adaptation (see the next section on sets and reps).

"So why then do we only deadlift once per week if we squat twice?"

Simple. The deadlift observably responds very well to being trained once per week (in both pure beginners and more sophisticated trainees alike), and the effects on overall recovery are skewed in a more favorable direction for the long haul since this program is designed to drive progress for a long period of time without the need to tamper with anything substantial (an ideal situation for the overwhelming majority of those reading this book). Again, a single five pound increase in the load lifted per week means a 20 lb gain over the course of the month, or 120 lbs in a six-month period, not too shabby if you keep the pace. Don't worry though; if you don't (which you probably won't and aren't expected to) there are other mechanisms built in to the plan by which you will be making smooth and steady gains.

"Why the A/B setup on the press/benchpress, and not on the squat/deadlift"

The press and bench press both use significantly less muscle mass than do the squat and deadlift. The resulting loads used for the former two lifts are smaller than the latter two, thereby placing less systemic stress on the body and its recovery ability. This allows one to train the two lifts in an alternating fashion each training session without any detrimental effects. Remember, the more opportunities for individual stress/recovery/adaptation (read: strength and muscle gain) cycles, the greater the potential for growth and strength development. We want to keep the frequency high and the load and the volume significant enough to elicit an adaptation, without providing an unnecessary beatdown that forbids us from getting back into that glorious growth cycle with another stimulus within the desired timeframe.

Section Two: Exercise Order

In this program I prefer to have the lifter perform the upper body lift (press or bench press) for the day first in the workout, before the lower body component. I feel that this allows for several advantages over doing the lifts in the reverse order.

Advantage 1: The lifter is freshest going into the first lift of the day. This allows for a lot of intensity to be applied to the movement as opposed to doing the lift after being fatigued from the previous lift(s). This is especially important when we are talking about attempting to follow the monster lifts, the squat and the deadlift with a lift like the press or the bench press. The most intense and grueling bench press workout you will ever have will not severely inhibit your ability to either squat or deadlift, while the reverse certainly is not true.

Advantage 2: As mentioned above, being fresh going into the first lift allows for a lot of focus and intensity in the movement. An observable phenomenon with demographics that use certain other linear progression models that feature the squat first is a relatively disproportionate level of development seen in the lower body, vs. the upper body, musculature. I have also addressed this issue in a number of other variables presented in this program, designed to facilitate the development of the most aesthetically balanced physique, out of the gate, as possible. That said, the simple adjustment of being able to train the upper body when it most fresh, and therefore capable of demonstrating the best performance against the weights, is enough in itself to make a noticeable difference.

Advantage 3: This approach allows the lifter to lay down and sulk for a few minutes after completing the very difficult squat or deadlift set(s) before heading home for the day, rather than worrying about having to get their mentally and physically drained body in gear to knock out the next exercise on the list.

Section Three: Sets and Reps

The floating, variable, reps in the Greyskull LP program are the first component of the 'periodization' element that makes it so effective. If one is locked into doing the same number of sets and reps workout after workout, it is obvious that they are going to hit a wall and need to do something to get past where they got stuck.

From here we will take a look at the sets and repetitions that are characteristic of this program.

What does 2 x 5, 1 x 5+ mean?

All of the lifts with the exception of the deadlift are performed for three total 'working sets'. This means that there is a series of warm-up sets (more on these later) and then three sets which are intended to provide the stimulus necessary to spur adaptation (the 'working sets'). The first two working sets are of five repetitions. The third set is taken to failure. This means that the lifter does not simply stop completing repetitions of the lift at five, or some other arbitrary number, but rather continues with the set until they are sure that the next rep will not be completed safely (as in the bench press or squat) or (as in the press or the deadlift) a failed attempt at a repetition is made.

Complete with warm-ups, a sample squat session may look like this (my notations are weight x reps x sets, and weights are in pounds):

Empty bar x 10 x 1

135 x 5 x 2
225 x 5 x 1
275 x 3 x 1
315 x 5 x 2, 315 x 7 x 1

The three sets at 315 lbs represent the working sets for that workout.

As mentioned before, the bench press and the press follow the same set/rep prescription that the squat does, so workouts of either of the aforementioned lifts would look similar in notation.

Sets and Reps for the Deadlift

The deadlift differs from the other lifts in both that it is only performed once per week in this program, and also in that it requires one hard working set. The single set used with the deadlift is similar to the final set in the other lifts, it is taken to failure and has no arbitrary maximum number of repetitions at which to artificially terminate.

A sample deadlift session, complete with warm-ups, may look like this (notations are weight x reps and all weights are in pounds):

135 x 6
185 x 5

205 x 5
225 x 3
265 x 9

Here the lifter gutted out nine good reps with 265 lbs before terminating the set, due to a missed attempt to pull the bar from the floor, or the belief that successfully lifting the bar would have required a deterioration of safe technique that was significant enough to warrant not risking the rep.

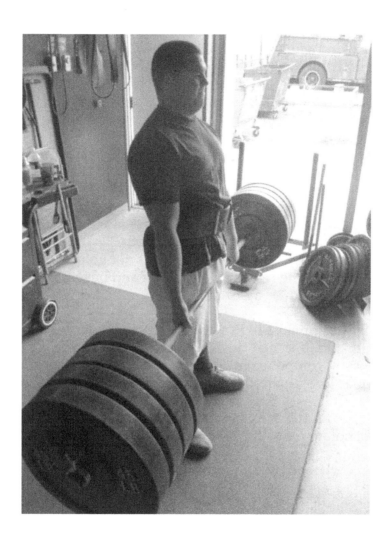

Section Four: Small Incremental Increases in Bar-Weight

As I touched on in the origins chapter, the pace at which the load being used on the barbell is increased is an important consideration when embarking on a weight-training program. It is important not to attempt to make greater increases in weight than one can successfully recover from and return to the next session stronger, and it is important not to come out of the gate too quickly. Being in too much of a hurry to hit a wall and get stuck or 'fry' the central nervous system by adding bar weight at unsustainable rates is a one way ticket to overtraining land. Some advocate starting with larger increases in bar weight at the beginning of a trainee's program, opting to reduce the increment as progress inevitably slows. This is not a terrible approach and works well. I, however, prefer to start the trainee out on a more realistic pace and make more conservative increases from the beginning, facilitating a longer stretch of time over which weight can be added to the bar. Often people are concerned that the smaller increases are a waste of time, and that since the trainee can handle the more stout increases early on why not use them? Again, this thinking is predicated on the idea that bar weight is the only variable in the equation, and that all sets are being performed for a fixed number of reps. Working within these restrictions, the above concerns are much more valid.

However when the sets are being performed to failure, the creation of a stimulus for growth and strength development is ensured regardless of the numerical value of the weight on the bar. Take a simple example: a man has a fixed barbell weighing 225 lbs. If he has a five rep max of, say, 300 lbs, performing a set of five with the 225 lb bar is not going to "knock anything loose" in the adaptation sense. However, if he reps the weight out and busts out a set of 17, with the last two being true ball busters, you can be assured that a stimulus was created.

Simply put working to failure, or close to it, with progressively heavier loads is going to make for a great deal of strength and muscular development. Though bar weight is not the be-all and end-all, it is still an important component of the whole picture and one should endeavor to drive it up as smoothly and for as long a period of time as possible.

It is for this reason that I opt for the use of smaller than average increases in bar weight throughout the program, not just once the going gets tough.

Standard increases from workout to workout for the lifts are as follows:

Squat and Deadlift: 5 lbs (or 2 kilos)
Press and Bench Press: 2.5 lbs (or 1 kilo)

The increases for the bench press and the press will require fractional plates, which can be purchased or improvised in order to make the required jumps in weight possible. *I cannot stress the value of acquiring or making these plates enough.*

A quick but important note on reps: When beginning the program, you will need to make an educated guess as to a weight that you will likely fail with at between eight and 10 reps. The last set (or working set in the case of the deadlift) is to be performed to failure, even if the set will be more than 10 reps. In the event that the set stretches out beyond 10, a decision is made as to whether or not to doulbe the increase in weight for the next workout.

For instance, in the event that a beginner squats 165 lbs for 17 reps in their first workout, they would be well suited to make a 10 lb increase at the next workout, in order to bring the reps in the last set closer to 10. If, instead, they were to get 12 or 13 reps they may opt to maintain the intended pace and just let the reps come down on their own from that point. This is less crucial admittedly on the squat, which responds very well to reps in the teens, but is much more of a concern with the pressing movements whose 'money' range is between six and-10 reps.

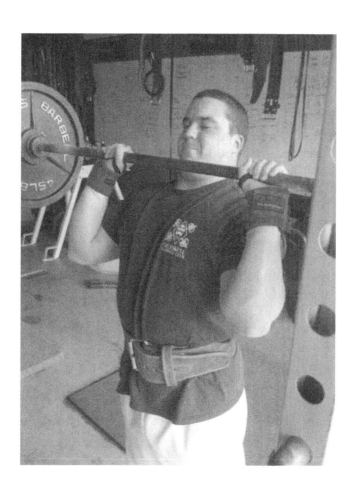

Section Five: The 'Greyskull Reset'; Enter the 'Periodized' Linear Progression

Ok, now we're going to get deep into the 'magic' that makes this thing so damned effective at getting people strong, and keeping progress going for long periods of time, without interruption or stagnation.

As I discussed in the origins chapter, in my opinion, the largest single flaw (there are a few) in the conventional linear progression-type model is how the 'reset' is handled, or what to do when the lifter is failing to make the requisite repetitions per set to warrant continuing to add weight to the bar. This program is set up to address that inevitable situation with a proactive and productive approach that will ensure the negative aura surrounding the reset in conventional programs is set out to sea. I really can't fault anyone for their negative associations, I mean who wants to take several steps back after working so hard to get to where they are? The trick is developing the association that the resets are an inevitable and tremendously valuable part of the program. We are not using bar weight as the center of our universe here, so it is just one variable.

The Greyskull Reset as applied to a bench press that has become stuck at 210 lbs would look like this (notations are weight x reps x sets, and all weights are in pounds):

First the lifter would calculate 10% of the bar weight, or simply work from the other direction and determine 90% of the previous working weight as the start point for the reset:

210 lbs x .9 = 189 lbs

I always have the lifter round down to the next nearest 5 lb (or 2 kilo) increment, so in this instance the starting weight would be 185 lbs.

The next several workouts may look like the following:

185 x 5 x 2, 185 x 11 x 1

187.5 x 5 x 2. 187.5 x 11 x 1

190 x 5 x 2, 190 x 10 x 1

192.5 x 5 x 2, 192.5 x 9 x 1

195.5 x 5 x 2, 195 x 10 x 1

Notice a few things:

-The weights were being increased by 2.5 lbs per session (this will require the use of fractional plates).

-The repetitions remained constant at 11 for the first two workouts. This isn't always going to be the case, but it should be the intention of the lifter to beat or at least tie the previous workouts rep max sets with the new, heavier weight each time they hit the gym.

-By the third workout, the repetitions on the last set started to decline. This is entirely normal, and is expected. The repetitions will drop as the weights increase over time.

-After managing 9 reps with 192.5 lbs the lifter was able to hit 195 lbs for 10 on his last set. This happens sometimes as well. It does not mean anything is wrong. It can usually be chalked up to an especially good workout due to any number of variables. Accept these when they happen, they are a good thing.

We'll rejoin our lifter now as he approaches the weight that he was unable to complete three sets of five with before…

205 x 5 x 2, 205 x 8 x 1

207.5 x 5 x 2, 207.5 x 7 x 1

210 x 5 x 2, 210 x 7 x 1!

Success! The lifter has now passed his sticking point and is breaking new territory again with the bar weight. He will continue to add 2.5 lbs to the bar each workout until he cannot successfully complete five reps on the last set. When this happens he will back the weight up by 10% and begin the reset process again.

This 'peaks and valleys' approach to loading is invaluable in its ability to allow a lifter to progress in strength and lean mass gain for quite a while without requiring any major program component be altered.

Here we will take a look at the reset approach applied to the single working set of the Deadlift:

315 x 4 (did not complete five rep minimum for last set, so time to reset).

315 lbs x .9 = 283.5 lbs

This means we will be using 280 lbs as the weight for the first workout. The following example illustrates how the following workouts may play out (remember, here we will be making 5 lb increases since we are deadlifting):

280 x 10
285 x 10
290 x 9
295 x 9
300 x 8
305 x 7
310 x 8
315 x 7

The above lifter is able to push past their previous sticking point, as well as set rep records at the lighter weights on the climb back up to new territory.

Let's assume the lifter in the case above makes it out to 335 before needing to bump it back again. With a conventional approach, 20 lbs of new territory may seem disheartening as an increase before a reset is needed. This type of thinking leads people to abandon ship on a program that would continue to work just fine if the resets were handled better.

Let's say in the first 'wave' the lifter gets stuck at 315. At that point he resets to 280 and gets 10 reps with that weight on his working set. The same lifter, being unable to complete five reps on his work set with 335 would take 35 lbs off of the bar for his reset, bringing the bar weight down to 300 lbs. In the first reset he was able to hit 300 for eight, how many do you suppose he will get this time remembering before he got stuck he was able to lift 330 for five, at least?

Let's be modest and say he squeezes 11 reps out at 300 this time around. Enough stimulus to build strength again, if he is capable of getting 335 for four? Absolutely.

How about muscle growth? Can you imagine 300 x 11 on the deadlift not being a good growth stimulus for this individual?

See where we're going with this?

The belief that bar weight is the only variable that can be adjusted is extremely limiting. The lifter may not be able to get the new PR bar weight for five, but the strength they've built on this cycle (the climb in weight and subsequent reduction in completed working set repetitions) will enable them to smash a lighter weight (which not too long ago *was* the PR working weight) for a PR in a higher rep range. This allows progress to be made **during** the reset. The overload idea is continued albeit through a different mechanism.

There's more than one way to skin a cat.

While we're on the subject, let's examine the conventional wisdom regarding rep ranges in regard to the specific adaptations they are traditionally considered to deliver?

Low reps with heavy weights for strength, high reps with lighter weights for hypertrophy, right?

We will get a bit more specific for our purposes here. Many sources agree that sets of five are ideal as a strength and mass builder, while lower reps are more suited for maximal strength, and higher than five rep sets are more for 'sarcoplasmic' hypertrophy, or the building of muscles that are 'all show no go'.

Too many take this idea too seriously in my opinion, possibly due to a body of scientific and anecdotal evidence. However, Can you imagine someone training only 12 to 20 rep sets on the squat and taking their working set of 12 from 155 to 315 lbs and not having more maximal strength, meaning a higher one rep max?

Dorian Yates and many other very successful bodybuilders long observed that certain rep ranges lend themselves very well to muscular development in certain exercises. For example, sets in the six to eight rep range (working at or near failure) were money for growth in the upper body pressing and rowing movements, while the Squat and leg movements in general seemed to work best with higher, double digit rep range sets. Additionally, single joint movements like curls and triceps extensions were most productive in the 12-20 range, near failure (no one wanted to tear a triceps tendon trying to use a huge three or five rep max poundage on a single joint movement.)

The single joint stuff I will touch on in a later chapter about add-ons, but at this point you are probably beginning to understand why structuring the program in the manner I have outlined; making incremental increases to allow continued progress in setting rep records (training near or at failure), and spending time hitting records from 12 reps or so on down to five with heavy loads is very conducive to developing a tremendous amount of muscular growth as well as getting significantly stronger.

A win-win situation; brute strength and muscular development in one program, with a stunning longevity rate in terms of your ability to make gains in both.

Chapter Three:
The Base Program

So now that we are familiar with the core ideas that comprise the Greyskull LP, let's take a look at the simple template for the application of the base program.

We are going to assume a Monday, Wednesday, Friday training schedule here in the first example, because it is probably the most common that I encounter among trainees, as well as for simplicity's sake. It should be implied that the days of the week do not matter so long as they (ideally) are not on consecutive days, and so long as there is a two-day break in the week at some point.

The three-day-per-week base program for two weeks will look like this.

Week One:

Monday
Press 2 x 5, 1 x 5+
Squat 2 x 5, 1 x 5+

Wednesday
Bench Press 2 x 5, 1 x 5+
Deadlift 1 x 5+

Friday
Press 2 x 5, 1 x 5+
Squat 2 x 5, 1 x 5+

Week Two:

Monday
Bench Press 2 x 5, 1 x 5+
Squat 2 x 5, 1 x 5+

Wednesday
Press 2 x 5, 1 x 5+
Deadlift 1 x 5+

Friday
Bench Press 2 x 5, 1 x 5+
Squat 2 x 5, 1 x 5+

This forms a solid foundation on which to build a program to achieve a wide variety of goals. With the primary strength-training component taken care of, the lifter can then tailor the rest of their training based on what it is they want to accomplish by 'downloading' the appropriate 'plug-ins' for their individual situation. The next chapter will discuss some of these additions, and how to implement them as part of a well-designed program.

The Base Program on a two-day per week schedule

Before we get into the plug-ins, we will take a look at the base program applied to two weight-training days per week. This is a common adaptation to the base program appropriate in several cases such as:

- A trainee with an erratic or demanding work schedule for whom three days per week is not possible due to other demands on their time
- A trainee who has family obligations that make training twice per week a more favorable option
- An older trainee who finds that they have difficulty managing the physical stress of training with weights more than twice per week
- A trainee whose wife/girlfriend or significant other is simply too hot and/or nymphomaniacal to make spending more than two days in the gym impractical (this one is a tragedy when we see it. I have had to cope with such stress for some time. All of you should feel bad for me.)

Whatever the reason, training two days per week is perfectly acceptable. It's true that progress in terms of building strength or lean body mass may not come as rapidly training less frequently, however it is important to remember that there are things in life infinitely more important than lifting weights.

As a matter of fact, stop reading for a minute and think:

Is strength training, or your time in the gym "your life"?

Is it what you live for?

If you answered yes to either of those questions please contact me at **john@villainintl.com** so that we can discuss this and get you on the path to a more meaningful and abundant life.

Ok, back to work. Here is a week of the Greyskull LP base program using a two-day schedule. In this case we are using Tuesday and Friday, but the training could obviously occur on any two days.

Tuesday

Bench Press 2 x 5, 1 x 5+
Deadlift 1 x 5+

Friday

Press 2 x 5, 1 x 5+
Squat 2 x 5, 1 x 5+

Simple and to the point.

Training two days per week in this manner will certainly produce results.

Chapter Four:
Building Your Greyskull LP: The 'Plug-ins'

In the last chapter we discussed the all-important foundation layer that the rest of the Greyskull LP is constructed upon. In this chapter we will examine some of the common things that we add to the base program to optimize progress towards particular individual desired outcomes.

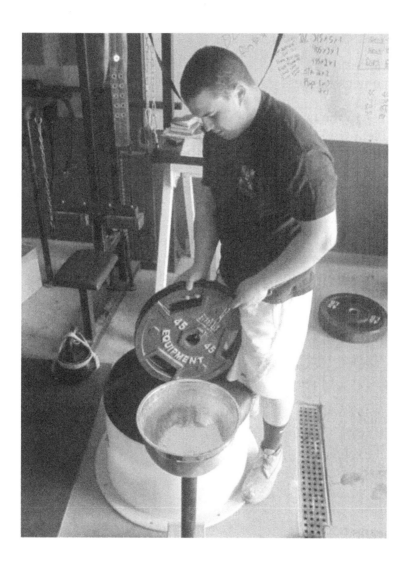

Section One: Additional Strength-Training Movements

One of the most common add-ons to the base program is the simple inclusion of additional strength-training movements.

The base program provides an extremely god foundation for strength and muscular development when left alone, however some have outcomes in mind that make adding some additional movements relevant.

In the first edition of this book I recommended three "standard" add-ons to the base program:

-Weighted chin-ups
-Curls (in different varieties)
-Neck extensions with a neck harness

These were included due to the fact that the versions of the Greyskull LP that I was writing about online generally featured these movements. At the time I was generalizing quite a bit in my writing; speaking to my primary audience at the time, males who were looking to build muscle and strength. The ideas were presented as a way to use a linear progression program that was more effective, and conducive to developing a more aesthetically pleasing body than what was commonly seen.

The principles of the Greyskull LP can be applied in designing a training program for a variety of different populations however; literally anyone that is looking to make serious progress and build strength can use the information in this book to do so.

That being said, let's look at some of the more commonly used additional strength-training movements.

- Curl Variants
- Neck Extensions
- Row Variants
- Chin/Pull-up Variants
- Olympic Lifts
- Direct Abdominal Exercises
- Direct Calf Exercises
- Forearm Exercises
- Pull-overs of
- Dips
- Cable arm movements

The above list is not all-inclusive. There are few rules on adding movements, the Greyskull LP is yours to do what you like with it, just remember that the base program will meet the majority of your needs. Adding additional exercises can help you accomplish certain specific tasks more efficiently, but you'll never go wrong by sticking to the base program by itself should you so desire.

Sets and Reps on the Additional Movements

I have few hard and fast rules when it comes to strength training, however, one that I am adamant about is not doing volume for the sake of doing volume. Anyone can subject a muscle to fifty reps or sixty reps of a movement during the course of a training session. I've always been more of a precision kind of guy. I don't want to carpet bomb, spray and pray, I want one shot, one kill.

What I mean by this is that I feel doing four sets of twelve, or five sets of ten of a movement after your main exercises for the day does two things:

For one, it forces you to use a weight that is far less than what you are capable of training with. Second, it promotes the idea that the movement being performed is an "assistance" or "accessory" movement, two terms that I hate.

Labeling the exercise with either of these distinctions implies that the movement is of lesser importance than other movements in the program. Imagine what that does for one's performance on the movement.

I am of the opinion that a curl should be performed with every bit as much attention, focus, and intensity as a squat. If you are choosing to include curls, or any other movement for that matter, for the purpose of affecting a particular adaptation, that movement should be considered every bit as important as the "big" lifts.

I'm not going to get into specific sets and reps for each of the above exercises. Recommendations for those will vary from individual to individual anyway, but I will provide a basic overview by movement that can help you determine an appropriate approach to incorporating these movements into your personal Greyskull LP.

• Curl Variants	Two sets: 10-12 repetitions
• Neck Extensions	Four sets: 25+ reps
• Row Variants	Two sets: 6- 8 repetitions
• Chin/Pull-up Variants	Two sets: 6-8 repetitions (if weighted)
• Olympic Lifts	5-6 singes per session
• Direct Abdominal Exercises	Two sets: 10-12 reps
• Direct Calf Exercises	One set: 15-20 slow, painful repetitions
• Forearm Exercises	Two sets: 12-20 repetitions
• Pull-overs	Two sets: 8-10 repetitions
• Dips	Two sets: 6-8 repetitions (if weighted)
• Cable arm movements	Generally in the 10-12 repetition range

These movements can be inserted into the training week as you see fit. Later, in the sample program section, you will see some examples of how I plug these movements into someone's schedule.

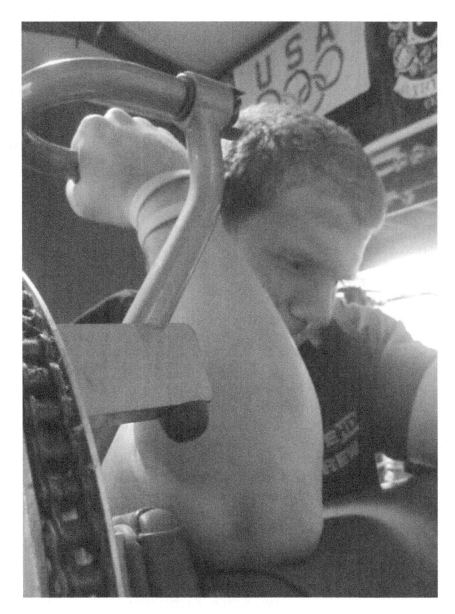

Greyskull Legend, "Biggs" pumping up on the Nautlius Curl Machine.

Section Two: The Frequency Method

The Frequency Method is a very effective technique for building muscular endurance as well as strength and size. It involves doing multiple sets, never to failure, throughout the day each day of the week (taking one completely off) and accumulating a ton of volume over the course of the week/month.

It is no secret that I loathe volume training when it comes to lifting weights, but with bodyweight exercises, volume is the only way to go. The biggest mistake people make when trying to improve on their bodyweight exercises while also getting stronger in the weight room is training the movements too intensely. I want you to leave nothing in the tank on the last set of the weight workouts, go for broke, every time. With the bodyweight stuff however, your work should always be 'easy'. Bodyweight exercises like chin-ups and push-ups in high volume are an excellent tool for upper body development. It is no secret that they are not as effective for said purpose as weight training, however I often say that there is an inverse relationship between the effectiveness of a given stimulus towards a specific adaptation and the frequency with which it can be applied. Therein lies the beauty of the Frequency Method. It can be used to layer in more work towards the goal of strength and muscular development without taking away from the weight training, and in fact acting synergistically with it, to produce and even better result.

The Frequency Method and the Chin-Up

Let's look at the Frequency Method as applied to the bodyweight chin up.

Let's say Pete can do seven good bodyweight chins at a shot. In his case, sets of four should be a breeze. We will begin by having him do six sets of four reps spread as thinly throughout the day as possible. He might do a set when he wakes up, one when he goes to bed (many are rigging chinning bars in their homes which I highly recommend) and then four more sets spread throughout the day when possible.

If he does this for 6 days the first week he will have done 144 reps total (24 reps x 6 days). The next week he may add a set and do seven total sets per day, or add a rep to his sets (assuming that the last rep is still **easy**, I can't stress this part enough). As long as you are doing a little more than last week you are doing it right.

Now let's say Pete can only do three good chins in one set. For him, the second rep of a set of three is probably starting to get tough. If this is the case, he will do singles, and add to the number performed per day sooner than he will add a second rep. So for instance...

Week 1: Seven to eight singles/day
Week 2: Nine to 10 singles/day
Week 3: Six sets of two
Week 4: Seven sets of two

By the fifth week he will probably be ready to start doing sets of three. He will know that he's ready if sets of two are very easy at this point. Each time the number of reps per set is increased, he should back up the number of sets per day by one or two. This goes for anyone at any level of ability, always step back a step or two when you add reps to your frequency method sets.

Frequency Method for Chin-Ups Alternative: The Ladder Method

The Ladder Method is our weapon of choice when the trainee cannot use the Frequency Method to its full potential due to scheduling reasons such as being stuck in an office with no access to a chinning bar all day.

A common mistake is to confuse the Ladder Method with the more conventional idea of doing a 'pyramid'. Let's look at the difference:

Two Ladders of three reps will look like this:

One set of one rep
One set of two reps
One set of three reps

Then repeat the same process beginning at one set of one.

One set of one rep
One set of two reps
One set of three reps

A Pyramid to three reps will look like this:

One set of one rep
One set of two reps
One set of three reps
One set of two reps
One set of one rep

The Ladder Method is greatly preferred over the Pyramid idea since it allows for better recovery during performance. The most difficult sets of the pyramid are clustered together at the apex of the pyramid, whereas with the Ladder, the hardest sets are followed immediately by the easiest sets. This allows for much more quality work to be completed in each session.

The number of ladders and the number of 'rungs' on the ladder will depend entirely on the individual and their ability to perform chins. The important thing here is that, like the Frequency Method, the top set of the ladder is not yet at the point where the last rep is extremely difficult. The idea here is accumulating a day's worth of volume in a short period of time; therefore the sets need to be relatively easy in order to make it through the ladder.

One can do ladders five to six times per week. The work is more concentrated than the work performed in Frequency Method sets since it is performed in one block of time instead of spread out throughout the day. This makes soreness and things like tendonitis (if they try to do too much too soon) an issue, especially for those just starting in this method.. It is important to gradually increase the work on these, and not make huge jumps in the amount of work being done per day/week. Start easy and add the days, reps and sets gradually.

A solid goal to strive for with chin-up ladders is five ladders of five reps. That's 75 reps in a very short amount of time. Work your way up to this point, then check in with me and tell me if you aren't happy with the upper body development and strength that you've gained in the effort.

"How long do I rest in between reps and ladders?"

The answer to this common question is **the amount of time it would take a partner to complete the set that you just completed**. Think of it like this, if you and I are doing a ladder tag-team partner style, you would knock out a rep and then I would follow suit. Your rest period would be while I was doing my work and vice versa. Maintain this pace throughout all of the ladders.If you can't keep up then you are doing much work for that day anyway, so reduce the number of reps per ladder, or drop a ladder, in order to make it more manageable.

So if you're doing this one by yourself you need to bring your imaginary friend along to help you pace yourself. Just make sure if you are doing this in a commercial gym or any other setting where you are not alone that you do not converse with your imaginary friend too loudly or people will think you're weird.

"But what if I can't do a chin-up yet?

If the trainee can't do a chin-up, then the first order of business is getting them the ability to do a chin-up. Once they can do one they can start using the frequency method to beef up their numbers (the first few weeks will be painful since they are operating near/at their max with each single, expect to see a temporary dip in performance on the upper body lifts during this time).

So how do we get them a chin-up?

The most tried and true method I've used over the years is the slow negative combined with progressively heavier v-handle pulldowns on a lat pulldown machine. Not everyone will have access to the latter piece of equipment, but anyone with a chinning bar can do slow negatives. The trainee simply gets himself or herself over the bar either with assistance or by stepping or jumping up. Then they lower themselves down until the arms are fully extended as slowly and controlled as possible.

At first they will more than likely sink to the bottom like the proverbial sack of shit. In time however, they will be able to control themselves much more and greatly control their rate of descent. This movement should be practiced often, frequency method style, though a word of caution must be given:

Negatives will make a new trainee very sore, so ease into them slowly.

Within a few weeks, unless the trainee is significantly overweight, they should be demonstrating the strength required to lower their body from the top to the bottom completely under control. At this point they should be very close to reversing direction and pulling themselves up over the bar. I promise you that if you are the trainer you will never have to tell them it is ready to try a full one. They will do it on their own when the time is right, and the two of you can share in the awesomeness of the first chin-up together.

If there is access to a lat pulldown machine, the pulldown can be used to build upper-body pulling strength that will greatly help in the quest for the first chin-up. I greatly prefer the v-handle to all other handles and find that it builds strength (and size where desired, hence its heavy usage in our Powerbuilding stuff) in a more direct manner than other variations.

The v-handle pulldown is performed for two sets of six to eight reps. This is done in lieu of the weighted chins on the pressing days in the base program (a practice which is continued until the trainee can do at least eight bodyweight chins), and in conjunction with the daily slow negatives. Like the weighted chin, the movement is trained rep range style, so the idea is to hit as many good repetitions as possible, which if the loading is correct should fall between six and eight. Once the rep range can be reached for both sets, it is ok to up the weight.

You may have heard the ridiculous arguments of some that the pulldown will not carry over at all to your ability to do pull-ups or chin-ups. I always found this comical. If someone comes in my gym and they can only get 90 lbs on the stack for six to eight reps for two sets and many weeks later they are doing sets with 260 lbs on the stack, do you honestly believe that they are not now significantly stronger? Many know someone who can do a lot of weight on the stack but is not a chin-up whiz. That's fine, that's because they don't *practice* chins. The secret here is that bodyweight exercises are a skill, and respond to frequent practice like any other skill (frequency method).

Now, do you suppose the real pulling strength earned on the stack will make it easier or harder to get good at doing a lot of chins?

I'll let you ponder that one for a minute.

Some are so jaded when it comes to machine use that they condemn their usage and therefore discourage many under their influence from ever experiencing the many possible benefits that machines have to offer. For the record I do not even consider cable stacks to be machines, and include them in the free weight category.

The Frequency Method and the Push-up

Now that we've dealt with the Frequency Method as it pertains to the bodyweight chin-up, we will take a look at the method in application to the simple push-up. The push-up is an excellent tool for developing upper body strength and muscle mass. A quick look at a cellblock will confirm this fact. It is no secret that push-ups are prison staples, and the boredom and motivation to train to build the suit of armor leads inmates to crank these out in high numbers all the time. Predictably this leads to some fairly impressive development as well as an athletic, battle ready vehicle.

As with the chin, one needs to stay well shy of failure with their Frequency Method push-up sets. For example, if Pete can do 30 good pushups before they start to break down, he should be starting with sets of 20 or so to start. Four or five sets per day for the first week will go a long way. Each week the number of sets, or reps per set, or both should increase if only by a small margin. The cumulative work from these will have a very positive effect on your physique as well as your pressing strength. Don't sleep on the value of these guys, add them in now and crank out easy sets of 75 in a few months (and then tell me how you look).

An excellent goal for a male trainee with pushups is Villain Challenge #3, completing 100 pushups in two minutes.

The Frequency Method and the Dip

A common question I get is whether or not you can do dips using the frequency method. The answer is obviously yes, but I would prefer you to be able to do a no-bullshit set of fifty pushups at the minimum before taking this on. Having a go at it before that point is much less productive. Same with more challenging exercises like handstand pushups. Get the pushups down first (at least 50 uninterrupted reps per frequency set), then the dips (at least 40 uninterrupted) then maybe the handstand pushups.

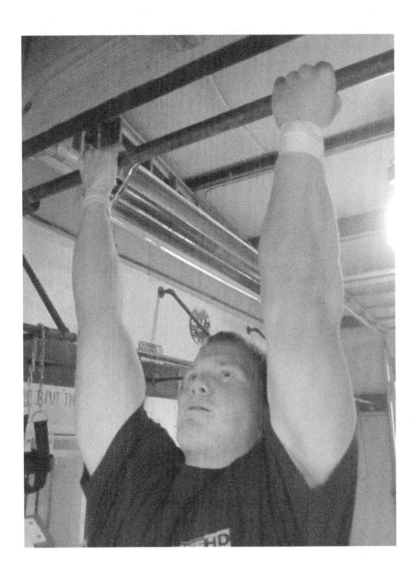

Bonus

Using the Frequency Method to Change your Body in Eight Weeks

A common technique that I have been using with consultation clients as of late involves building simple daily habits that compound and lead to tremendous gains in a short period of time. When I discuss the 'Blueprint to Beast' success formula[2] with private clients we identify three components:

- Standards
- Beliefs
- Habits

The first two we will not be getting into here, however we will take a quick look at how we can build a habit that will deliver huge success in a short period of time.

Let's take the example of a male trainee who desires an aesthetic more in line with that of Jason Statham (we share a hair-do).

I might inform this client that in order to install a habit one must simply perform an action everyday for twenty-one days.

Three weeks. That's it.

Make yourself do it for three weeks and you own it.

Now, here's the trick. We keep the work in the initial stages very easy. This way the trainee does not associate pain with the activity and continues to do it each day as scheduled. By the time the activity becomes challenging, it's already installed as a habit.

So let's say that we build a habit of performing a chin ladder, and a push up ladder each night at home. A doorway chin up bar or some other apparatus is all that is needed to do this.

---

[2] Blueprint to Beast is a proprietary system of personal development methods that I teach in seminars, consultations, and in a multimedia package later this year. If you're interested in learning more about how to use the Blueprint to Beast material to achieve success far beyond your expectations, contact me at john@villainintl.com

It would look like this:

- Monday   Chin Ladder
- Tuesday   Push-up Ladder
- Wednesday   Chin Ladder
- Thursday   Push-up Ladder
- Friday   Chin Ladder
- Saturday   Push-up Ladder
- Sunday   Chin Ladder

That's right, every day. Keep the total reps per day down, increase gradually, and never to the point that you are near failure during any set.

What might you predict the trainee's result may be after eight weeks of this uninterrupted? Would they look more or less like Jason Statham would you say?

How much time per day would they need to invest in order to make this happen?

What do you suppose would happen if we added burpees (Villain Challenge 1 layer) with the ladders each day?

Did you notice how we did not discuss diet once during this, yet you know somehow that the trainee's body would adapt favorably and look different in spite of whatever dietary practices they had?

Can you imagine what would happen if we added weight training three days per week on top of this, coupled with a solid diet? An unfair advantage huh?

Is there any possible way this would not work to deliver tremendous progress?

Food for thought huh?

And now my favorite question:

What are you waiting for?

Section Three: High Intensity Conditioning

This particular layer is the one that probably causes the most controversy. There is a common misconception that one cannot train to get bigger and stronger while also training to become more athletic and/or to improve their body composition. This thinking dictates that in order to get big and strong you first have to become fat and strong.

Well, not really.

We aren't going to be touching on the nutrition side of things in this book, but I will let you in on the secret that you do not have to take in gross amounts of calories from shit foods and gallons of milk in order to grow muscle mass. I definitely acknowledge the fact that there needs to be a caloric surplus in order for there to be growth (my track record is fairly respectable in terms of packing muscle on trainees) but nowhere is it written that this has to be accomplished with poor food choices and in such excess that the boobs and belly are grown more than the back and bi's.

In addition to not needing to eat like a video game kid with a tapeworm, one need not abandon everything resembling anything athletic in order to grow either. What good is being strong if you look like a barrel ass and can't walk up a shallow grade without becoming a sweaty, disgusting mess? That's not what my clients want and that's probably not what you're after as a reader.

Fact of the matter is, one can lift weights three days per week with intensity, knock out Frequency Method sets of bodyweight exercises, and perform multiple conditioning sessions per week if they're smart about it with zero detrimental effects.

In order for this to work two main points need to be taken into consideration:

-The trainee must be eating enough
-The conditioning workouts need to be short and intense

The first one we aren't going to get into in this book, but the second point we will touch on briefly. In order for the work to make sense and fit nicely with the base program and its other plug-ins, the sessions need to be very intense and short in duration. In my books '50 Greyskull Approved Conditioning Workouts for the Modern Viking', and it's sequel, aptly titled '50 More Greyskull Approved Conditioning Workouts for the Modern Viking' (both available through Villain Publishing in the store at StrengthVillain.com) I talk about the '10 minute rule'. This simply refers to 10 minutes being about the maximum amount of time one of your conditioning sessions should last without it being excessive and getting into the territory of shitting on the rest of your training and/or generally beating you up to the point that the other aspects of your training cannot be hit with the appropriate amount of intensity to drive progress.

The above-mentioned books showcase 100 examples of workouts used here at Greyskull that fit this mould well and can be used as an integral part of a well laid out Greyskull LP.

Initially I will recommend one add two of these high intensity conditioning sessions to the training week, ideally one after the Wednesday (assuming a Monday, Wednesday, Friday lifting schedule) session, and one on Saturday as a stand-alone event. If desired, a third session can be added after a week or two on one of the other training days.

Hit these hard and reap the benefits of being a big, strong, athletic beast, a member of Greyskull's "Nation of Linebackers" (a term I borrowed from my good friend Anthony Roberts).

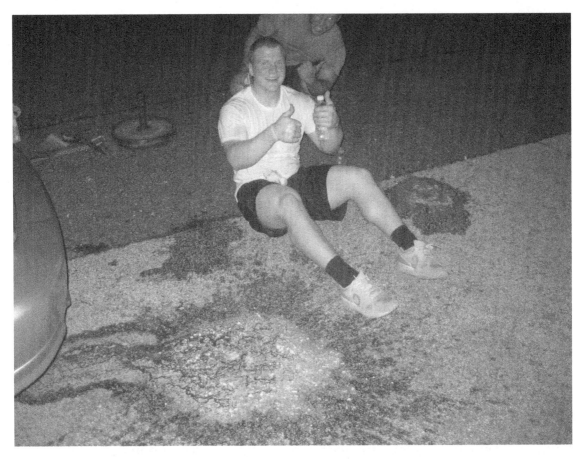

It happens to the best of us. 'Biggs' after creating the vomit equivalent of the Great Lakes, with Bony approaching, chloroform in hand, behind him.

Section Four: Low Intensity Conditioning

This is by far the lamest of the plug-ins, but it is damn effective in shedding body fat, hence its frequent inclusion in programs that I write. It is certainly not the type of activity that the average hard charging strengthvillain.com reader gets all fired up about participating in, but do not skip over this section if you were not blessed with a naturally low level of body fat regardless of how you train or what you eat, and do not want to look like a bar league bowling champion instead of a lean, muscular, hulking personification of Astroglide.

The concept here is simple, the tool even simpler. The preferred method for low intensity cardio is fast walking.

Yep that simple, and yep, that boring.

So if we like intensity so much in our weight training and in our conditioning sessions, why do we want to do the least intense activity possible, and on top of that, why would we want to do this type of activity with the greatest frequency out of all of the other tools?

Let me further pique your curiosity by making the statement that low intensity conditioning is not very effective at burning body fat at all…

… in a single application, that is. Therein lies the rub.

It is interesting to note that there is an inverse relationship of sorts between the efficacy of a given stimulus in producing a desired adaptation and the frequency with which that stimulus can be administered.

For instance, when it comes to building a strong, lean, body, weight training is king. There is no better activity that you can engage in to get you closer to the goal of a strong body with a great body composition than weight training. However, if you are training with the requisite intensity necessary to produce the type of adaptation desired, you must necessarily limit your exposures to the weights to a maximum of three sessions (with few exceptions allowing for a fourth). A good way of looking at it is that you need to have more recovery days per week than you have weight training days since it is during the recover from weight training not during the activity itself that you develop the strength and muscle mass.

The Frequency Method is great for building muscle and to a somewhat lesser degree strength, yet due to the lack of intensity involved relative to the intensity needed for effective weight training (enhanced by the fact that we deliberately avoid going to failure or even near it in our sets), the method can be applied many more days per week than its more intense and more effective cousin weight training. Once a person is acclimated it is not at all uncommon to see Frequency sets occurring five to six days per week. This 'layering' of stimuli in terms of its relative position on this 'hierarchy' is precisely what enables one to use these various methods with a synergistic effect, rather than having them negate the effectiveness of each other or greatly tax the overall recovery capability of the entire system.

It's true that higher intensity conditioning burns more calories than low intensity work, both in the immediate application and through the EPOC (Excess Post-Exercise Oxygen Consumption) phenomenon that allows the metabolism to stay ramped up for hours after the event. This is frequently cited in the marathoner versus the sprinter example. We must necessarily limit the exposures to the higher intensity work however if we hope to make solid gains in a consistent and predictable manner in the weight room (which will in turn add muscle which brings with it an increased resting metabolic rate and ultimately a greater ease in getting and staying lean, more proof of how weight training is the most effective tool for transforming your body). This is where the chronically-applied low-intensity work comes in to shore up the excess taken in through the diet needed to pack on the muscle, and work on eliminating the reserves through a passive aggressive means that consumes primarily body fat as fuel over other available fuel sources (this last part is precisely why this method works best when fasted and glycogen depleted [carb cutoffs anyone?] first thing in the morning).

Simply put, if there was a more tried and true, effective manner of losing body fat while maintaining - if not gaining - new muscle mass every bodybuilder and physique competitor on the planet would be using it. Ask them what they do to get lean (besides strict diet) and you will get a chorus of 'lots of cardio' by which they mean consistently applied low intensity, muscle sparing, fat burning work. It is important to note that the pre-contest phase for a bodybuilder (with or without the aid of drugs) is typically 16 weeks in duration. That's four months! This speaks to the value of consistency of effort over long-ish periods of time.

The great part about this tool is how simple it is to apply. Most everyone in the world can walk and it requires no special equipment. If you're trying to get leaner, work on layering in the low intensity sessions, walking quickly for anywhere from 20 minutes to an hour, preferably fasted, first thing in the morning, as many days per week as you can handle. Lather, rinse, repeat over time and watch the fine lines come out in the mirror.

Bonus

A Tried and True Fat Loss/ Conditioning Tool for Commercial Gym Cardio Equipment

This is a cardiovascular training method I borrowed from Bill Phillips, author of 'Body for Life' and other titles years ago. I have experienced great success using this method on a treadmill, elliptical trainer, or recumbent bike.

Well over a decade since I first read about this training method, I still apply it with trainees on a regular basis. It serves as an excellent bridge between the worlds of high and low intensity conditioning, and is very effective when used consistently as a part of a fat loss program.

Bill Phillips called it the "Twenty-minute Aerobic Solution"; you'll call it the balls for shedding the fat off of your frame.

The Twenty-Minute Aerobic Solution

This method requires the use of a perceived exertion scale, a concept that may be new to some readers. It is much easier than it sounds. The scale simply requires that you assign a number, from one to ten, to the amount of effort that you are putting forth. A lower number reflects a lower level of exertion.

For instance in the case of an in-shape trainee, a five might be a somewhat brisk walking pace, while an eight would be a hard run, and a ten would be an all-out sprint.

A one might be simply standing up, make sense?

Good.

Ok, so now that you understand how this number scale works, let's look at how to use this information to trim the fat

The workout will last twenty minutes. Each minute of the workout will have an exertion level associated with it. This method can be used successfully on any piece of commercial gym equipment.

Elliptical trainers and Recumbent bikes offer more freedom in terms of pushing hard during the more demanding minutes, though I tend to prefer the treadmill for it's "set it and forget it" capability; once you crank it up to the desired number you have no choice but to keep the intensity there.

Minute	Intensity Level (one through ten)
1	5 (warm up)
2	5 (warm up)
3	6
4	7
5	8
6	9
7	6
8	7
9	8
10	9
11	6
12	7
13	8
14	9
15	6
16	7
17	8
18	9
19	10 (all out effort)
20	5 (cool down)

Section Five: Villain Challenge #1; The Burpee Layer

This particular add -on is one of my favorites. It is the one 'elevator conversation' tip that I have given more people, both of the training variety and those met in social situations who weren't accustomed to training, that has provided me with the most predictably positive feedback besides "basically just stop eating sugar all together for six days out of the week". Its simplicity is remarkable and the assumption by which it works makes it seem almost too easy.

Basically here it is:

Villain Challenge #1 (which can be seen on strengthvillain.com along with the other villain challenges) involves being able to complete 100 burpees in five minutes. This is no easy task, as anyone who has ever tried it will tell you. The interesting part is the simple correlation between body fat percentages and one's ability to perform this task, read:

I have never seen someone complete this task that was unsatisfied with his or her body composition.

Does this mean that one can simply diet their body fat down and they will magically be able to knock this challenge out, or that someone with a naturally low body fat percentage will have little difficulty in nailing this?

No.

What it does mean is that if someone sets out to achieve this goal, and trains for it specifically, , they will invariably end up happy with their body composition on the day that they knock out this challenge.

Am I saying that the burpees themselves are magic, and that they incinerate fat when done for a few seconds every day?

No, I'm not. In fact, I'm not making any claims as to the efficacy of the burpee for fat loss. All I am saying is:

I have never seen someone complete this task that was unsatisfied with his or her body composition.

This ties in with the question I often pose to people "How many chubby 11 second 100m dash sprinters do you see?"

Point is, if you set a performance goal that requires the development of a great deal of athleticism, chances are that you are going to look like you possess a great deal of athleticism when you reach your target.

Here is an overview of how I have trainees train for this one.

Performing 100 burpees in five minutes requires you to maintain a one-burpee-per-three-second pace. The trick is to gradually increase the number of burpees that you can do while staying on pace.

Most will be fine to start out with three sets of 10 reps. In this case you would have a 30 second window within which to knock out each set. In the beginning the rest in between sets can be several minutes if need be, but you should endeavor to reduce the rest in between efforts down to one minute over time.

Once you can perform the target number of reps in the target amount of time, you are ready to add reps. These mini workouts are to be done daily (six days per week) so you should add the reps very slowly, one or two per day to ensure that you are not outpacing yourself. **Increase the amount of time allowed for each set by three seconds for every rep that you add.**

Once you can do sets of 30 in 90 seconds or less, each with one-minute's rest in between, you are ready to reduce the number of sets to two and keep pushing the number of reps per set up. Once you can do two sets of 50 in less that two and a half minutes each, you are ready to start doing one single set each day, gradually pushing towards the ever elusive 100 rep mark.

Stick with this one (many do not) and be one of the few that commits to accomplishing this goal. I promise you will not be disappointed in the least with the outcome of your efforts.

Chapter Five: Putting it all Together
Applications for The Greyskull LP

You will notice the similarities in structure and implementation of the base program, but will also be able to observe the individual differences that are made to skew the adaptations in a particular direction. Understand that these are merely examples and are not written in stone. Individual differences often warrant addition or subtraction of layers to/from the program in order to facilitate the optimal training conditions for the trainee, so keep that in mind when viewing these.

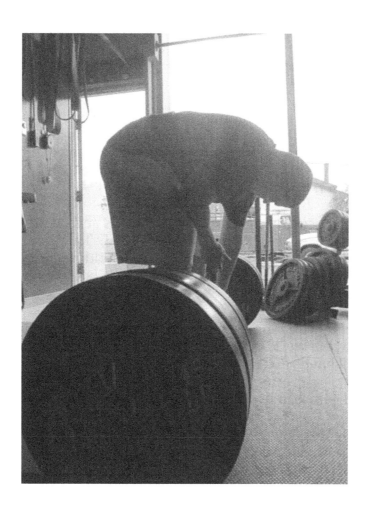

The Greyskull LP for Mass Gain

I have used the principles outlined in this book to personally add a significant amount of muscle mass and strength to my body numerous times over the last several years. More importantly, I have used these principles very successfully to add the same to hundreds of people worldwide. Combine that data with that of the thousands that have been influenced by the information on the GSLP available on the Internet, or who have purchased the eBook online and you're left with a critical mass of evidence that suggests that the Greyskull LP is the balls when it comes to building size and strength.

So how do we use the information in this book to add muscle mass?

Well, for starters, muscle mass and strength have enjoyed a long-standing relationship. In simple terms building strength in a progressive manner using big, compound barbell movements remains King in terms of adding muscle mass to one's frame. I will qualify that by saying that a diet conducive to that adaptation is required as well, which we will be discussing a bit in a minute.

Big gains in strength equal big gains in muscle mass when the body is fed accordingly. We understand that the Greyskull LP in its most common form is a heavily barbell oriented, strength-training program that consists mainly of compound movements. It is therefore a no-brainer to understand why the principles in this book applied in conjunction with a solid mass-gain diet make one hell of a recipe for packing on the beef.

Increased caloric intake, particularly from protein rich foods and quality carbohydrates, is key to adding lean body mass to one's frame. In my book: "SWOLE: The Greyskull Growth Principles", I outline the ideas that I use in building mass building diets for my clients for which that is the desired outcome. I highly recommend reading the book if you're intent on adding mass to your frame.

So think about it, a male trainee eating beef and rice, drinking protein shakes mixed in milk, lifting weights three times per week using the GSLP principles, and using AM walks as his primary conditioning will have what predictable result?

If you said that he would gain lean body mass you are correct, give yourself a pat on the back.

The mechanics of the weight-training program can be used in a strikingly interchangeable manner to reach desired outcomes. The variables such as diet and additional "plug-ins" are much more responsible for how the results are manifested.

Here are some examples of actual Greyskull LP programs I've written for others with a mass gain focus.

Modified Greyskull LP Mass Gain Base with Rotating Lifts

Monday

Incline Bench Press: 2 x 5, 1 x 5+
Curl Variant: 2 x 10-12
Squat: 2 x 5, 1 x 5+
Neck Harness: 4 x 25

Wednesday

Press: 2 x 5, 1 x 5+
Weighted Chin: 2 x 6-8
Yates Row: 2 x 6-8
Deadlift: 5+
Neck Harness: 4 x 25

Friday

Decline Bench Press: 2 x 5, 1 x 5+
Curl Variant: 2 x 10-12
Front Squat: 2 x 5, 1 x 5+
Neck Harness: 4 x 25

Here we see several of the lifts being rotated.

The bench press movements are alternated between incline and decline, and the squats are alternated between back squat and front.

The idea behind this is that each lift progresses for a longer period of time, while two or more different stimuli are being used concurrently as part of the same program. There are infinite ways of laying out a Greyskull LP program using this idea.

Greyskull LP with Mass Gain/Strength and Hypertrophy Focus

Monday

AM: Fasted walking (20-30 min)
Throughout day: Frequency Method Push-ups and Chins
PM: Weight training
Press 2 x 5, 1 x 5+
Weighted chins 2 x 6-8
Squat 2 x 5, 1 x 5+
Neck harness 4 x 25

Tuesday

AM: Fasted walking (20-30 min)
Throughout day: Frequency Method Push-ups and Chins

Wednesday

Throughout day: Frequency Method Push-ups and Chins
PM: Weight training
Bench press 2 x 5, 1 x 5+
EZ curl bar curl 2 x 10-15
Deadlift 5+
Neck harness 4 x 25

Thursday

AM: Fasted walking (20-30 min)
Throughout day: Frequency Method Push-ups and Chins

Friday

Throughout day: Frequency Method Push-ups and Chins
PM: Weight training
Press 2 x 5, 1 x 5+
Weighted chins 2 x 6-8
Squat 2 x 5, 1 x 5+

Greyskull LP with Greyskull Gladiator "Linebacker" Focus

Monday

AM: Fasted walking (20-30 min)
Throughout day: Frequency Method Push-ups and Chins
Burpee workout (VC 1)
PM: Weight training
Press 2 x 5, 1 x 5+
Weighted chins 2 x 6-8
Squat 2 x 5, 1 x 5+
Neck harness 4 x 25

Tuesday

AM: Fasted walking (20-30 min)
Throughout day: Frequency Method Push-ups and Chins
Burpee workout (VC 1)

Wednesday

Throughout day: Frequency Method Push-ups and Chins
Burpee workout (VC 1)
PM: Weight training
Bench press 2 x 5, 1 x 5+
EZ curl bar curl 2 x 10-15
Deadlift 5+
Neck harness 4 x 25
High intensity conditioning session

Thursday

AM: Fasted walking (20-30 min)
Throughout day: Frequency Method Push-ups and Chins
Burpee workout (VC 1)

Friday

AM: Fasted walking (20-30 min)

Throughout day: Frequency Method Push-ups and Chins
Burpee workout (VC 1)
PM: Weight training
Press 2 x 5, 1 x 5+
Weighted chins 2 x 6-8
Squat 2 x 5, 1 x 5+

Saturday

Throughout day: Frequency Method Push-ups and Chins
Burpee workout (VC 1)
High intensity conditioning session

The Greyskull LP for Fat Loss

The Greyskull LP principles are incredibly flexible with regard to the adaptations that they are able to produce. We've already discussed the appropriateness of the Greyskull LP for building lean body mass, now let's look at the other side of the body composition coin; fat loss.

When using the Greyskull LP principles for fat loss, as with a mass gain program, the diet and the "plug-ins" are what make the magic happen so to say.

In order to trim the fat, attention needs to be paid to the diet. There is much room for discussion of this subject, most of which is outside the scope of this book, but suffice to say that an understanding of food quality, portion sizes, meal timing, and what constitutes a solid meal needs to exist if one is to be successful.

I have long been a proponent of emphasizing feeding the body for progress, then shoring up any excess caloric intake with activity rather than using a gross restriction of calories.

This "activity" driven approach has worked wonders for me over the years, and has lead to a great deal of people achieving results they previously though unattainable.

Some basic diet tips to apply when fat loss is the desired outcome are as follows:

- Drink only calorie-free liquids
- Eat protein with every meal
- Choose protein sources that are low in fat primarily (think chicken or fish over beef)
- Eat smaller, more frequent meals throughout the day
- Use vegetables (preferably raw) to "fill up" on during meals
- Read labels and otherwise be aware of what you are taking in macronutrient and calorie wise from your foods

The diet portion of a fat loss program can obviously get much more complex than the above, but those ideas will certainly provide a head start to a motivated, driven individual who is applying the information in this book to change their body composition.

The Fat Loss "Plug-ins"

Activity is key with fat loss, plain and simple. Burn up more than you are taking in, and you will lose fat.

Choosing plug-ins to layer into your GSLP that are conducive to dropping the fat is critical if you are to succeed.

The "big three" that I make use of when laying out a program for someone with fat loss in mind are

- Low Intensity Conditioning (preferably fasted)
- High Intensity Conditioning (Find out loads of examples in my books "50 Greyskull Approved Conditioning Workouts for the Modern Viking, and the sequel "50 More Greyskull Approved Conditioning Workouts for the Modern Viking" The "Twenty Minute Aerobic Solution" can fall into this category as well
- Villain Challenge #1 Progression (the single most effective, yet under-utilized fat loss tool I know of)

Let's have a look at three sample programs written for people with fat loss as a primary objective.

Run Forrest, Run

Monday

AM Fasted Walk: 30-45 min
Press: 2 x 5, 1 x 5+
Squat: 2 x 5, 1 x 5+

Tuesday

AM one-mile run

Wednesday

AM Fasted Walk: 30- 45 min
Bench Press: 2 x 5, 1 x 5+
Deadlift: 5+

Thursday

AM sprints: 100m x 8

Friday

AM Fasted Walk: 30-45 min
Press: 2 x 5, 1 x 5+
Squat: 2 x 5, 1 x 5+

Saturday

5k run

Sunday

Off

Commercial Gym Fat Loss

Monday

AM Fasted Walk: 30-45 min
Press: 2 x 5, 1 x 5+
Squat: 2x 5, 1 x 5+

Tuesday

20-minute Aerobic Solution (see page 47)

Wednesday

AM Fasted Walk: 30-45 min
Bench Press: 2 x 5, 1 x 5+
Deadlift: 5+

Thursday

20-minute Aerobic Solution

Friday

AM Fasted Walk: 30-45 min
Press: 2 x 5, 1 x 5+
Squat: 2x 5, 1 x 5+

Saturday

20-minute Aerobic Solution

Sunday

Off

Four-Day Beast Split

Here we see the base program lifts limited to one per day, and spread across four weight-training days.

Monday

Squat: 2 x 5, 1 x 5+
Sprint: 100m x 8
VC 1 Progression

Tuesday

Bench Press: 2 x 5, 1 x 5+
Dumbbell Front Squat, Push Press, Squat and Press x 35
VC 1 Progression

Wednesday

VC 1 Progression

Thursday

Deadlift: 2 x 5+
100 yd Bear Crawl x 4
VC 1 Progression

Friday

Press: 2x 5, 1 x 5+
"13 Down" Ketllebell Swing/ Burpee (see 50 Greyskull Approved Conditioning Workouts for the Modern Viking)
VC 1 Progression

Saturday

One-mile run
VC 1 Progression

Sunday

VC 1 Progression

In this case, the Villain Challenge #1 progression is done every day because the person is tasked with doing it every day for three weeks in order to install it as a habit.

It should go without saying at this point that there is room here for the trainee to add extra work such as frequency method bodyweight exercises. These are merely sample templates, like everything in this book, there is nothing about them that is set in stone.

The Greyskull LP and the Female Trainee

A common question that I receive is whether or not the GSLP is appropriate for a female trainee. The simple answer is yes, of course, but there are certainly some considerations and adjustments that can be made in order to better suit the needs or wants of a female.

First, as we have previously discussed, there is no single, "correct" version of the Greyskull LP. There are only backbone principles that form a foundation for which the program is built uniquely for (or by) the individual.

Common questions I receive by some less-informed as to what the GSLP actually is by definition include:

"Do you have females do the neck harness?"

"My wife/girlfriend doesn't want to do curls, what should I do?"

"I've had great success in gaining some serious muscle mass using the Greyskull LP. My wife wants train with me, but she doesn't want to get bulky, what do you recommend?"

Understanding that the program is simply a set of principles that can be applied with flexibility to the individual case allows us to answer those questions rather easily.

With regards to the neck harness: I include the neck harness "plug-in" in most of the programs written for males for a few reasons, not the least of which is the desire to create a larger, stronger neck. In all of my experience, I have only encountered one female who was hell bent on increasing her neck size.

The simple answer is no, I don't have females use the neck harness.

It's not a part of the foundation of the program, but merely one of the more commonly used (by males) plug-ins.

Same with the curls; more women are interested in doing curls than training their neck, but the majority I encounter are not interested in any additional arm development beyond the firming and "toning" that naturally comes with performing the main barbell exercises that are typically associated with the base program. The reality is that the curls are included for increased arm development for those who are interested; they are not in any way mandatory in order to reap benefits from training with the Greyskull LP.

The idea of a woman not "bulking up" from this program or any other is a topic that has been discussed a great deal elsewhere, and most that are reading this book are probably already familiar with the reasons why weight training won't turn a woman into the hulk. Just in case the reader is brand new to this however, I will address the simple reason why this isn't possible.

Women are not hormonally capable of developing man-like muscles. The Flex magazine beauties that have scared women away from weight training for years are not passing a drug test any time soon.

Simply put, unless a female is using steroids, she will not develop a man-like physique. Now, that said, what can a woman expect?

A female interested in embarking on a personal development journey, using the Greyskull LP as the foundation for the physical component will experience some certainly favorable adaptations.

The use of barbells and other strength training tools in a progressive manner to build strength will develop the muscles that give their body it's womanly figure. The difference in the silhouette of a man and a woman is most directly attributable to the muscle on their skeletons, hence why a woman who is anorexic or otherwise malnourished lacks the physical features that are associated with femininity. Imagine a starved man (or one who's done CrossFit for too long), and a Hollywood female who's been in the news for becoming a mere skeleton standing next to each other, hard to discern who's who from a silhouette alone, isn't it?

Frankly, lifting weights and strengthening muscle makes a woman look *more* feminine, not less.

"Firming" and "Toning"

Women often speak of wanting to "tone" this or that, or "firm" up a bit. "Tone" is a result of the amount of stored tension in a muscle, its readiness to perform tasks. Basically the stronger a muscle, the firmer it is to the touch.

This means that developing strength is the fast track to "firming up".

Stronger muscle also means a higher resting metabolic rate, more good news for the female looking to trim the fat. Combine the 'round the clock effects of an elevated metabolism from strength training with the direct fat burning effects of intense conditioning work such as wind sprints, and the frequent use of callisthenic movements to provide a slow and steady benefit. What you end up with is one hell of a recipe for a lean, firm, attractive female body.

Coincidentally you also have a solid description of how I lay out programs for females using the Greyskull LP principles.

Here are a few examples of possible GSLP programs for females:

Commercial Gym Setting/ Fat Loss/ "Toning" focus

Monday

AM: Fasted Cardio Session- 30 min Elliptical Trainer
Press 2 x 5, 1 x 5+
Squat 2 x 5, 1 x 5+

Tuesday

AM: Fasted Run ~3 miles
Chin Negatives- 6 with one-minute rest in between

Wednesday

Dumbbell Bench Press 2 x 5, 1 x 5+
Sumo Deadlift 5+
Kettlebell Swing x 150 (timed)

Thursday

Chin Negatives 6 with one-minute rest in between
Zumba class every other Thursday with friends

Friday

V-Handle Pulldown 2 x 6-8
Leg Press 2 x 10-12

Sat

Fasted Walk- 45-60 minutes
Push-up Ladder 3/5/7

Sun

Off

As you can see in this particular variant, some of the movements have been changed due to capabilities in the environment, the commercial gym in this case. Minor adjustments to the rep schemes are also seen depending on the movement used.

There is a three-day schedule used, yet there is no upper-body pressing movement on the third weight training day. In this case, the hypothetical female is not terribly interested in upper body development, but is more concerned with leaning out, and firming/developing her legs and butt. The sumo deadlift was the go-to here for that purpose as well.

You also see a variety of conditioning stimuli being used. There is fasted machine cardio, fasted walking, running, and high-intensity kettlebell work all being used in the same training week. This adds variety, keeps things exciting, and, in this case, fits in with this particular woman's work and family schedule.

The Essentials (Strength Focus for sport)

This female actively participates in a women's soccer league and is in great physical condition. Her body is solid; aesthetics are not a primary concern for her. Her largest reason for training with the Greyskull LP is the development of raw strength to make her better at her sport.

Here we stay remarkably simple. Her sport practices are omitted from the layout, all you are seeing is her strength training.

Monday

Incline Bench Press 2 x 5, 1 x 5+
V-Handle Pull down 2 x 6-8
Squat 2 x 5, 1 x 5+

Tuesday

Off

Wednesday

Press 2 x 5, 1 x 5+
Chin Ladder to 3, 3 times
Power Snatch 5 singles to warm up Deadlift
Sumo Deadlift 5+

Thursday

Off

Friday

Incline Bench Press 2 x 5, 1 x 5+
Squat 2 x 5, 1 x 5+

Saturday and Sunday

Off

Aggressive Female Fat Loss

Monday

AM: Fasted walking (40-60 min)
PM: Weight training
Squat 2 x 5, 1 x 5+
Press 2 x 5, 1 x 5+
High intensity conditioning session

Tuesday

AM: Fasted walking (40-60 min)
PM: Low intensity conditioning (20-40 min)
Burpee workout (VC 1)

Wednesday

AM: Fasted walking (40-60 min)
PM: Weight training
Bench press 2 x 5, 1 x 5+
Deadlift 5+
High intensity conditioning session

Thursday

AM: Fasted walking (40-60 min)
PM: Low intensity conditioning (20-40 min)
Burpee workout (VC 1)

Friday

AM: Fasted walking (40-60 min)
PM: Weight training
Squat 2 x 5, 1 x 5+
Press 2 x 5, 1 x 5+
High intensity conditioning session

Saturday

AM: Fasted walking (40-60 min)
PM: Low intensity conditioning (20-40 min)
Burpee workout (VC 1)

Sunday

Off

Two-Day Per Week Butt Developer Program

Here we have a woman who is interested in training in the husband's garage gym, primarily for the purposes of adding some much needed ass development. The husband has the basic home gym equipment for the famous "Linebacker" version of the GSLP outlined in the first edition. She is new to lifting weights and only wants to commit to training twice per week in the evenings, after dinner.

Tuesday and Thursday nights will be the strength training nights. There will be an effort made to walk or run in the neighborhood two other days out of the week.

Wind sprints will be run as a family affair on Saturday mornings.

Tuesday

Push-up Progression Work
Squat (High Bar position) 2 x 5, 1 x 5+

Thursday

Chin Negatives 5 singles with one minute rest in between
Sumo Deadlift 2 x 5+

The above represent four examples of the Greyskull LP principles being used in four different cases, and looking entirely different in each application. These examples by no means represent the only variations of the GSLP available to a female, but rather demonstrate the flexibility of the principles that make up the program.

It would be entirely possible, for example, for a woman who was training in a garage gym as in the third case to perform a routine more similar to the woman from the first case while keeping the lifts basic in nature to make use of the available equipment. Likewise, our soccer star could train twice per week in a commercial gym.

As I've stated throughout the book, there is nothing set in stone when it comes to training effectively. It is important to begin with an outcome in mind, and be flexible in approach on the road to seeing it through. The ability to tailor the program to the individual's desires is incredibly important, and is what any high-performing coach will be able to do. The ideas presented in this book are every bit as applicable and flexible for a female as they are for a male.

The Greyskull LP framework serves as an excellent program for a female looking to make positive changes in an efficient and enjoyable manner.

The Greyskull LP for Powerlifting

I am commonly asked how one can adapt the principles in the Greyskull LP to training and preparing for a Powerlifting meet. The simplest thing to remember is that the Greyskull LP is a strength-training program, and a very effective one at that, so the trainee is being prepared in a general sense for a powerlifting competition from day one.

I have maintained for years that Greyskull Barbell Club is not a powerlifting gym, yet numerous members over the years have competed, and performed well, in meets in various federations. We've held state and national records in a few weight classes in certain federations as well. It is important to note that the lifters who took home those titles for Greyskull did not train specifically for the purpose of increasing their one-rep-max in any lift, but rather to increase strength in general.

A stronger trainee always means a stronger one-rep-max.

One common adjustment that I make to the programs of trainees who are interested in competing in powerlifting is reducing the reps per set that are acceptable before the reset is necessary. By this I mean that instead of the trainee resetting the load once they are unable to perform five repetitions in the last set, I will have them continue increasing the load until they are unable to make three repetitions in the last set.

This acclimates the lifter better to handling heavier loads on a regular basis.

Training the squat in this manner for four weeks might look like this:

Week One

Monday Squat Session: 305 x 5, 5, 6
Friday Squat Session: 310 x 5, 5, 5

Week Two

Monday Squat Session: 315 x 5, 5, 4
Friday Squat Session: 320x 5, 4, 4

Week Three

Monday Squat Session: 325 x 3, 3, 4
Friday Squat Session: 330 x 3, 3, 4

Week Four

Monday Squat Session: 335 x 3, 3, 3
Friday Squat Session: 340 x 3, 3, 2

Week Five

Monday Squat Session: Off
Friday Squat Session: 305 x 5, 5, **10**

You'll note a few things that are a bit different about this set up.

As you can see, on Monday in week two, the lifter was unable to make five reps on the last set. At this point weight was added anyway, and the next session went on as scheduled.

When the lifter was unable to make five reps on two of the three sets, the reps in the first two sets were reduced to three.

If this method is to be used, continue to perform five repetitions per set on the first two sets until you are unable to complete five reps on any two sets. At that point, reduce the repetitions in the first two sets to three and continue performing the maximum number of repetitions possible on the last set.

You will also notice that there is an off day scheduled on Monday of week five. This is the first scheduled session after the reset has taken place when the lifter is unable to complete three repetitions in the last set on Friday in week four.

Always take a day off from the lift being reset after failing to complete the requisite number of repetitions on the previous workout.

This simple technique will allow the lifter to come back and make significant gains again, beginning with the conventional five, five, rep max scheme as seen in the Friday session in week five. Here the lifter managed ten repetitions with 305, a weight that they had only been able to handle for six reps in week one.

The ten-rep set demonstrates the strength that has been built in the last four weeks.

"Peaking" for a Powerlifting Meet

Peaking is a concept that I am often asked about as it pertains to a lifter using the Greyskull LP principles to prepare for a powerlifting meet. As I mentioned before, I train my lifters to build strength first and foremost, outstanding performance in competition is simply a byproduct of that approach.

Not unlike the method outlined in the previous section of reducing the reps required in the last set prior to reset however, I do make a few adjustments to one's training if I know that they are preparing to compete.

For one, beginning six weeks out, I will have the lifter begin taking some heavier weights after completing their work for the day.

This would look something like this:

Week One (of six leading up to meet)

Monday Bench Session: 275 x 3, 3, 5 290 x 2
Friday Bench Session: 277.5 x 3, 3, 5 295 x 1

Week Two

Wednesday Bench Session: 280 x 3, 3, 4 300 x 1

Week Three

Monday Bench Session: 282.5 x 3, 3, 2 *No additional lifts
Friday Bench Session: 255 x 5, 5, 9 300 x 2

Week Four

Wednesday Bench Session: 257.5 x 5, 5, 8 305 x 2

Week Five

Monday Bench Session: 260 x 5, 5, 8 310 x 1
Friday Bench Session: 262.5 x 5, 5, 8 310 x 2

Week Six

Wednesday Bench Session: 265 x 5, 5, 5 305 x 2
Saturday Meet Day Bench: 305, **315**, **320**

Ok, so let's look at what happened here.

Beginning in week one, I had the lifter take a heavy double after completing his work for the day. It was not a two-rep-max, but rather a very hard effort, in this case 290 x 2.

After the Friday workout, I had the lifter up the weight and get 295, this time for a single.

In week two we saw the lifter make a 300 single after his work, this was intended to be a double, but he just didn't have it in him that day.

In week three's Monday session, the lifter missed his requisite reps, demonstrating more of the fatigue that caused him to miss his challenging, but doable, 300 double the week two. I pulled the plug and reset him. There was no heavy attempt on that day.

Week four saw the lifter go back to higher rep work, and smash an easy 305 double.

In week five I pulled him back to a single at 310 after his work, which he easily managed. On Friday I had him repeat the weight for an easy double to gain confidence.

On week six, he adapted his normal Wednesday session so as to only perform the minimum five reps on each of the three sets, and then took his scheduled opening weight for the meet for an easy double. Emphasis was placed on this day on pausing the bar at the chest in accordance with the rules of the federation he is to compete in.

On meet day he took an easy 305, set a new personal record with an easy 315, and grinded out 320 to complete the day.

Not bad work at all.

Understand that there is no set-in-stone formula for determining what the correct number of repetitions (single or double) to have the lifter perform after their work. You can see that it varied in this case. What is important is that the work for the day is done. The additional rep(s) are just practice for game day, the real strength is built during the scheduled session.

The Greyskull LP for Olympic Weightlifting

Another common question that I am asked is how to modify the Greyskull LP to incorporate training for the Olympic lifts, the Snatch, and the Clean and Jerk.

I am not by any means the most accomplished coach of these movements, or competitors competing in them, however, I have enjoyed great success in training individuals to higher levels of performance in the lifts while continuing to get globally stronger, and, most importantly, enjoy themselves in the process.

Here are two examples of how the Olympic Lifts can be practiced and trained while Greyskull LP principles.

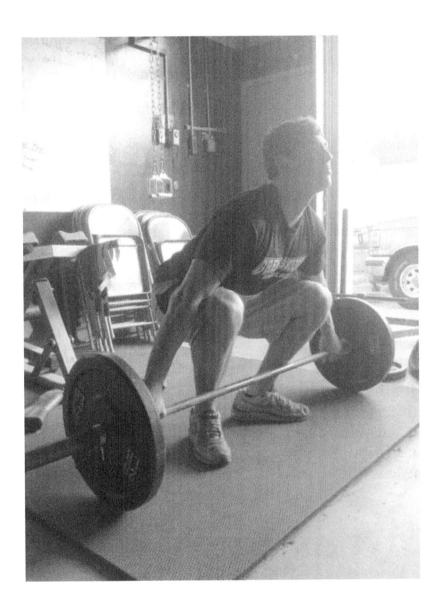

The "Luke Version"

One of the forum members on Strengthvillain.com once inquired about how to train the Olympic Lifts while using the Greyskull LP. I wrote him out a simple version of what I would recommend in a case like his and aptly dubbed it the "Luke Version". Not a great story, I know, but whatever.

Monday

Snatch: 7- 10 singles with ~ one minute rest in between (there is no set percentage of 1RM or anything being used here, just stick to a weight that is challenging, but that you can make unless you exhibit some sort of obvious technique blunder. You need to practice making lifts, not missing them)
Press: 2 x 5, 1 x 5+
Squat: 2 x 5, 1 x 5+

Wednesday

Bench Press: 2 x 5, 1 x 5+
Power Clean: 5- 6 singles ramping up to weight to be used for the Deadlift (hit 3 or so "heavy reps")
Deadlift: 5+

Friday

Clean and Jerk: 7- 10 singles (following same guidelines as Monday's Snatch workout)
Press: 2 x 5, 1 x 5+
Front Squat: 2 x 3, 1 x 3+

Obviously other layers could be added, conditioning work, frequency method, etc. This is simply to demonstrate how the base would be modified in this case.

Joshie's Limeade

This one comes to us courtesy of my good friend, and former Pan Am games competitor Josh Wells. He's not much of a dancer, but he's good at helping people become better weightlifters.

Monday

Bench Press: 2 x 5, 1 x 5+
Squat: 2 x 5, 1 x 5+
Row Variant: 2 x 6-8

Wednesday

Snatch: 6-10 singles (10 the first week, 6 the second)
Clean and Jerk: 6-10 singles (6 the first week, 10 the second)
Front Squat: 3 x 3

Friday

Press: 2 x 5, 1 x 5+
Squat: 2 x 5, 1 x 5+
Deadlift: 5+

Chapter Six: Exercise Index

Simplicity: An Introduction to the Greyskull Approach to Coaching Movement

"Before I studied the art, a punch was just like a punch, a kick just like a kick. After I learned the art, a punch was no longer a punch, a kick no longer a kick. Now that I've understood the art, a punch is just like a punch, a kick just like a kick. The height of cultivation is really nothing special. It is merely simplicity the ability to express to the utmost with the minimum."
-Bruce Lee

There is a lot of money to be made in making things a lot more complicated than need be. This practice of making things "proprietarily complex" as I like to say, is rampant in the strength and conditioning industry. Despite the fact that people in gyms all over the world with little to no training in the proper execution of exercises use them daily with great success, there exists a crippling belief in many that performing a proper squat or deadlift requires a textbook the size of a Philadelphia phonebook to learn from.

This belief is propagated largely by those who make money off of overanalyzing human movement and presenting their "findings" to skinny-fat internet surfers who know much more about training than the "bench and curl" meathead at Gold's Gym, but who, almost without fail, fall horribly short to the meathead in terms of aesthetics, strength, athleticism, desirability to the opposite sex, frequency of sexual activity, or any other metric more valuable than one's comprehensive knowledge of the biomechanics of the squat.

Simply put. You do not need an advanced degree in human biomechanics to successfully apply (or coach, yes I said that) the movements outlined in this book.

It is necessary to understand movement to the extent that you are capable of executing an exercise in a manner that will not produce injury, and which will be productive in terms of developing strength. Beyond that, most of what takes place on message boards in terms of "form" or "technique" analysis amounts to little more than the actual masturbation that takes place in front of the same screen after logging out of the strength forum.

The single biggest difference between those who do big things and those who do not is that those that do big things DO big things. No amount of reading, or watching videos on strength training will teach you more about the subject than getting off your ass and actually training.

If anyone were to contest that idea (and there are plenty that do publicly or internally) would have to agree at the very least that it is impossible to make physical progress without actually taking action at some point.

A common experience shared by many of my consult clients looks something like this.

- Start training with little knowledge
- Experience noticeable, exciting progress in aesthetics and strength
- Develop an interest in training from the momentum created
- Research and learn more about biomechanics, programming, and diet
- Progress comes to a halt
- Blame halted progress on program, end of some sort of stage of adaptation, diet, or some other mechanical component that is not the cause
- Contact me out of frustration
- Re-discover simplicity after learning how limiting beliefs cripple our progress
- Divorce limiting beliefs
- Make significant progress again
- Enjoy training again
- Make continual progress

Overanalysis of this stuff will get you nowhere. This is the reason why people who post on the StrengthVillain.com forum looking for a "form check" from me get such simple answers. I give them one item to fix that will have the most significant impact on the movement globally, then request another video if I deem it appropriate. What happens almost across the board when I do this is the follow up post from some other knowledgeable and well-meaning forum member providing insight on the mechanical issues that I somehow missed.

What needs to be understood is that I DO see those things, I just do not care that they are happening. "Correcting" them will do nothing more than add more items for the individual to consciously focus on while performing the movement that they would have gotten strong using "incorrectly" had they not contacted me or logged into the Internet anyway.

I can almost hear the internal dialogue:

"How does Johnny Pain not see him doing X?"

"His eyes/ears/ knees/ etc. are not in the right spot, how is it JP doesn't see this?"

And then inevitably:

"Wow, JP really isn't that good of a coach at this stuff".

I recently had a conversation with a StrengthVillain.com forum member who has become a friend over the last several months. The topic of coaching the barbell lifts came up (OK, you know for a fact I did not bring that shit up) and he began naming a who's who of "internet coaches" informally ranking them in terms of who was the best coach.

My name was surprisingly low on the list. I lost much sleep over this as you can imagine. To this I simply asked what constituted his criteria for a good coach. His eventual answer had much to do with a "coaching eye", an invaluable skill for a coach to have, and an in-depth, comprehensive knowledge of the movements presented.

I suggested that the best coach was simply the one who was most capable of eliciting reproducible results in line with the desired outcomes of the individual being coached.

Perhaps this was my way of making the rules work in my favor (my track record of delivering plus one for my clients is pretty damn solid), I don't know, but I do know that the ability to deliver is what I look for in a good coach.

Delivery requires communication.

Communication requires acutely tuned senses and flexibility.

Neither of these things require exhaustive laboring over biomechanical texts that you could beat (or bore) someone to death with.

Presenting an idea in a sentence is better than a paragraph and represents a much clearer understanding of the information by the communicator. Presenting in a paragraph is admittedly better than a page, and a page is certainly better than a novel.

Consider the process of learning a foreign language in high school. There is a formalized lesson plan, a textbook, homework, quizzes, tests, projects etc. Recall the process of working through verb conjugation charts and translating lists of vocabulary words. Now ask yourself if you are as competent of a communicator in that language as a nine-year old child who grew up in an environment where that language was spoken, received no formal education in it whatsoever, and has used it daily since.

Of course you aren't.

Learning a skill does not require textbook, or even a formalized instructor. The perceived dependence on said people or materials in order to make progress is a significant handicap of the informed trainee.

The information presented regarding the execution of the movements in the following section is deliberately simple. It is without complex, anatomical descriptions of the musculoskeletal components involved, and similarly devoid of the idea that there is only one acceptable model for the movement's execution.

Now,

You can chalk this up to my lack of knowledge, or you can attribute it to my having come "full-circle" and learning that a kick is a kick, a punch is a punch.

Enjoy.

Bonus Section

Breath Control for Lifting Weights

Breathing is an important part of lifting weights correctly in order to maximize result, and prevent injury. It is however, an often-neglected component of the mechanical side of things.

There's an excellent "rule of thumb" that I use in coaching clients in the proper execution of the lifts. It is incredibly simple:

Do not breathe while a barbell or other strength-training implement is in motion.

Abiding by this rule eliminates much of the need for further coaching on breath control.

It is also important to note that it is critical to take a large, full breath prior to performing a movement.

Think: "Bigger the movement; bigger the breath"

The squat for instance requires that a gigantic breath be drawn in and held prior to the descent. No breathing takes place until the lifter is back to the upright position at the completion of the movement. A long, slow, lung-emptying exhalation is not what is needed at the end either, but rather a short "push" of air out through the mouth to make room for another gulp of air to be brought into the lungs prior to the next repetition.

In smaller movements such as the press or bench press even, there is not a definite need to exhale and top off the lungs in between each rep. It is common, and often times preferable to execute more than one repetition while holding the same breath in the lungs. This is something that tends to occur naturally as a lifter progresses in experience. I do not emphasize developing this skill when coaching new lifters, but do not discourage it if I see them begin to do it on their own.

So basically, to recap;

Don't breathe if a bar is in motion.

Fill up your lungs before executing any lift.

The bigger the movement the bigger the breath.

The Squat

The Squat has long been regarded as the King of all Barbell lifts. It is without a doubt one of the most effective lifts in terms of building strength and muscle mass, the latter being dependent on the other variables necessary for growth being in place. It is a vital component of a well-designed strength-training program, and it is my opinion that all able-bodied individuals who endeavor to acquire more strength should be squatting.

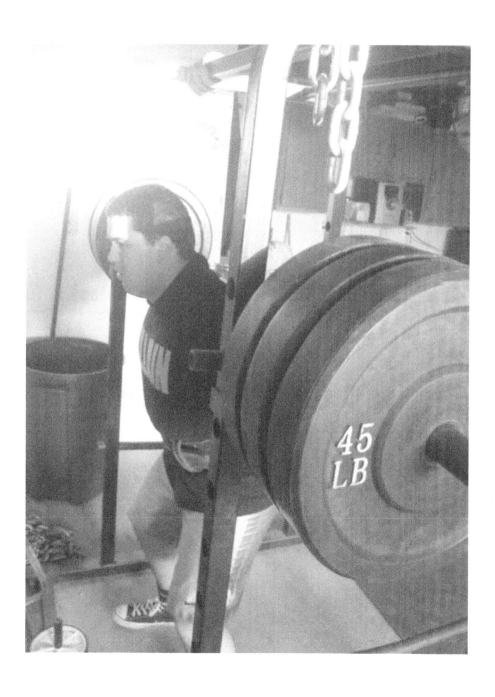

I feel that people commonly make teaching the squat significantly harder than it really is. I have developed a very simple method for teaching the squat that I have had tremendous success implementing with new trainees, and even experienced trainees who were grossly over thinking the movement prior.

With the bar placed on the back in a position that is comfortable for the lifter (as shown below) the lifter assumes a stance that will facilitate a proper squat. There will be a great deal of variance in terms of foot placement from person to person based on a variety of anthropometrical factors. There are however some "constant" characteristics of a good squat stance that can be modeled to shorten the learning curve.

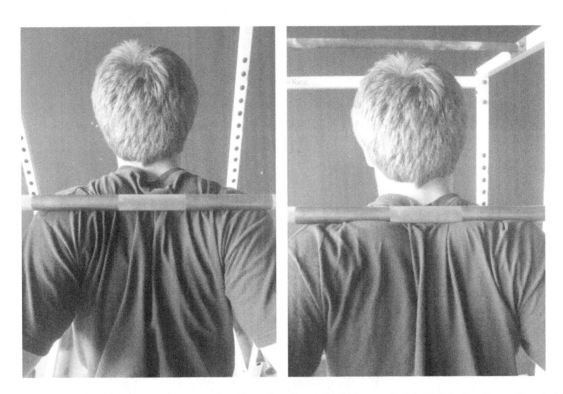

The two major "styles" of bar placement; the "low-bar" on the left, and the "high-bar" on the right. Either method is acceptable in my book. The rest of the movement remains the same from a teaching and execution standpoint. Squatting produces result, period. A prime example of minutia b.s. impeding one's progress is the nonsensical belief that a two-inch difference in the placement of the bar on one's back determines whether or not the movement is effective.

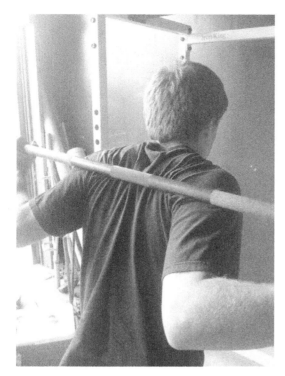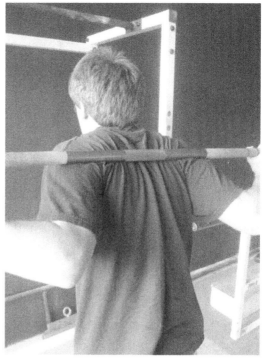

An over-zealous "low-bar" squat. Here the bar is too low, and is resting on the back of the arms. This is incredibly common with the "thumbs on top" method of holding the bar. Your elbows will hate you for attempting this.

For one, the feet will be turned out slightly. We aren't going to break out the protractors here and determine an angle, largely because of the great deal of variance in angle from person to person, instead we are going to instruct the lifter to turn his or her feet out slightly, and then let them surprise us with how much innate ability they have to position their own skeleton in a manner that will best allow it to move and function effectively.

Spacing of the feet will vary as well, however, placing the heels roughly under the shoulders will work for the overwhelming majority of the population, male or female.

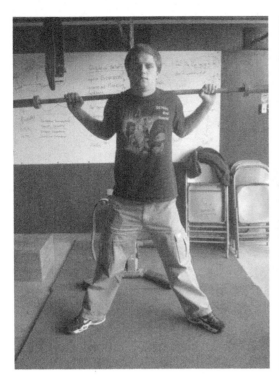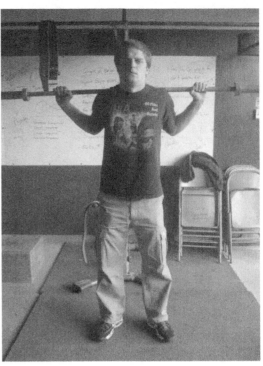

On the left we see Joe assuming a stance that is too wide. On the right we see a stance that is too narrow. In both we see a fly-ass NWA shirt.

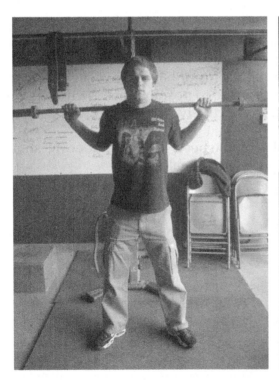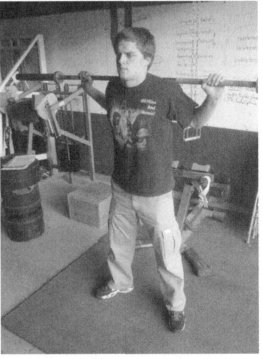

In the above images we see Joe in a stance that is just about right for him. Note the angle of his feet and the placement of his heels roughly under his shoulders.

Once we have the bar placed on the back with the hands around the bar (where it will be our instinct to place them) and we have assumed a proper squat stance, we are ready for the rest of the method.

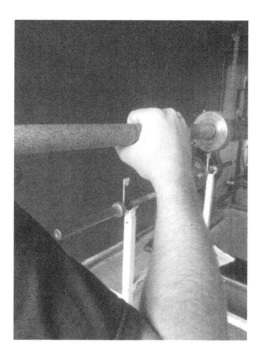

Do this

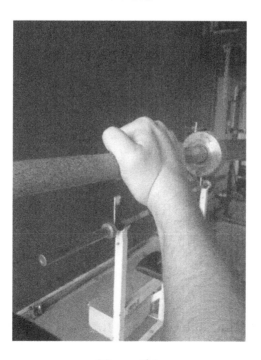

Never this

A well executed, balanced squat can be had by performing the following three tasks simultaneously:

1. Push the chest out as hard as you can,
2. Push the butt straight back as hard as you can
3. Push the knees out laterally as hard as you can
4.

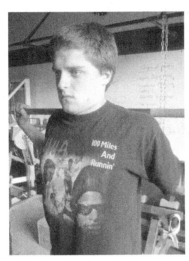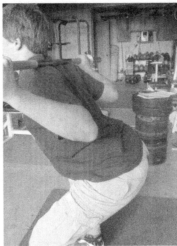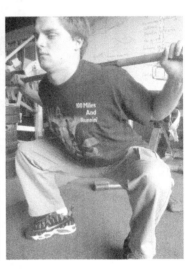

Chest out, Butt out, Knees out!

If all three of those tasks are accomplished simultaneously throughout the duration of the movement, the squat will always be performed in balance, with the bar riding in a prefect groove over the center of the foot.

Bonus Section

Correcting Common Squat Faults Using this simple Method

Interestingly enough, I have been able to successfully correct virtually any common squat fault by cueing one of the above actions.

For instance, someone who is having the bar come forward and sacrificing depth on the squat due to a rounding of the upper back (or caving of the chest depending on your perspective) who is familiar with this method can be cued to a fix by my simple vocalization of the word "chest".

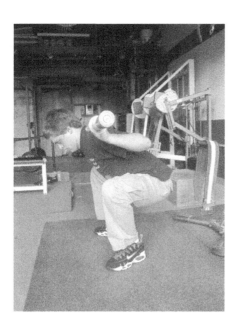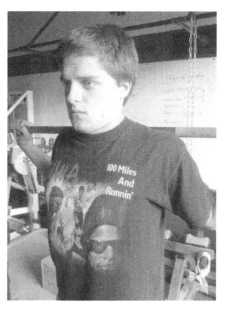

Here, Joe is demonstrating what takes place when a lifter rounds their upper back in the squat. Note how the bar is positioned in front of the mid-foot. This is a common problem that is exacerbated by the head down, elbows up position taught by some. Focusing on the chest out hard component fixes this. The lifter need only be cued with the word "chest".

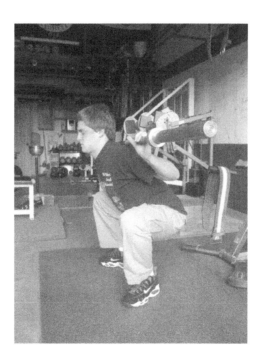

The result; a corrected bar path.

A lifter who is "down squatting", as I call the practice of attempting to place one's butt on the heels, neglecting to sit back, will have their knees come progressively more forward as the squat gets deeper. This will in turn cause the bar to come forward of the balance point over the center of the foot, and pull the entire system off balance. This common fault is corrected by simply saying, "butt".

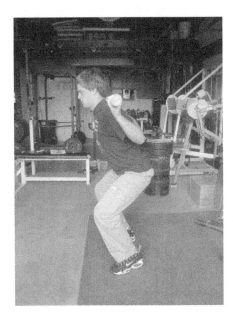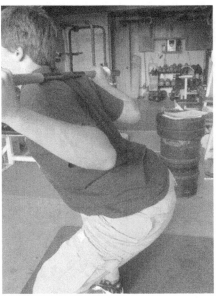

In the image on the left Joe is performing the common squat fault I call "down squatting". His knees are too far forward as a result of trying to "sit his butt on his heels". This is corrected by emphasizing the butt back portion of the method. He would be cued by simply saying, "butt".

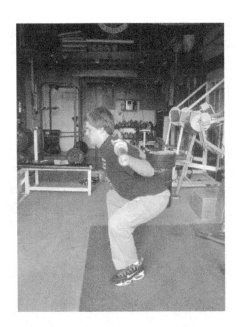

The result: A corrected bar path on the descent.

Inadequate depth in the squat is commonly caused by not pushing the knees out to the sides enough to allow the torso to pass between the legs. There are dozens of pages that can be written about the anatomical reasons for this, suffice to say that it is a common problem, and an extremely simple condition to remedy. The fix for this fault is predictably emphasizing "knees".

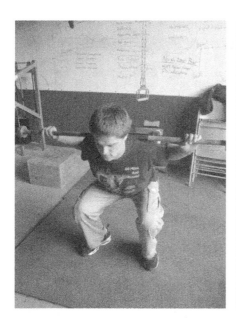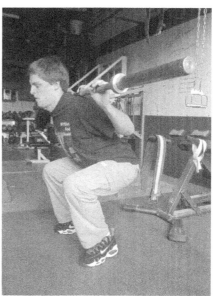

In the above photos we see Joe failing to push his knees out, causing an inability to get adequate depth in the squat.

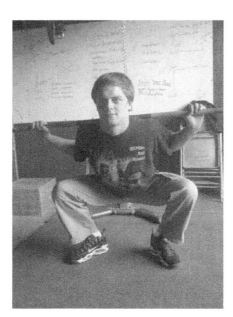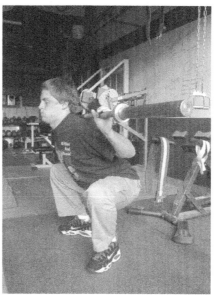

Joe focuses on pushes out his knees as hard as possible when cued "knees", the result; a deep squat.

This method takes the commonly overcomplicated task of teaching or learning the squat and makes it dramatically simpler. Less time spent over-analyzing the movement or arguing about it on the internet (a practice that is certain to induce celibacy) means more time to squat, get stronger, and build muscle, the purpose of performing the movement in the first place.

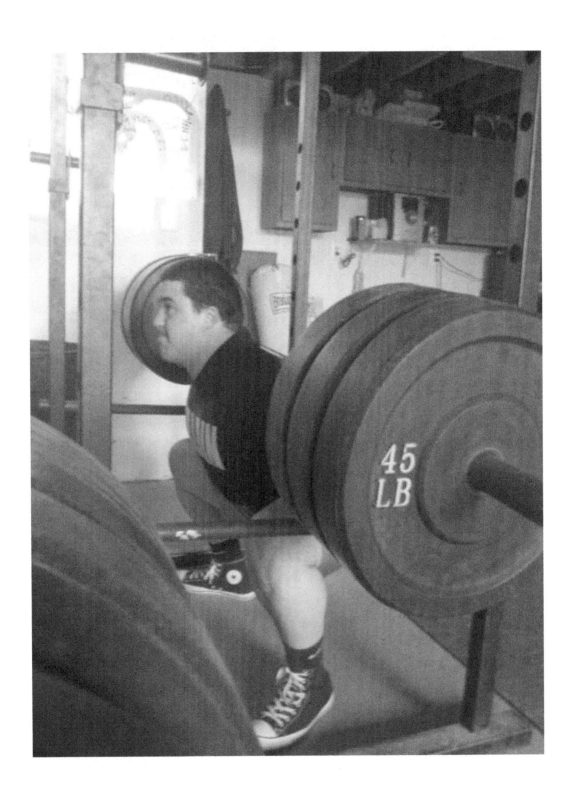

The Deadlift

The deadlift is the brother lift to the squat. Together they make a hell of a one-two punch in terms of building global strength. The deadlift, like the squat, should be included in any solid strength-training program.

Performing the deadlift is quite simple. It involves picking a barbell up off the ground, an action that every human has performed with other objects since they were old enough to do so. Despite the inherent ability that human beings have to use instinctive mechanics to pick up a load in this manner, many seek to complicate the performance of the lift by over-emphasizing the all-unimportant details of its execution.

Let me qualify this by saying that it is necessary to understand how to execute the lift "correctly" in terms of reducing the risk of injury, but beyond that there is not much of a difference between the technique of a beginner, and the technique of an accomplished deadlifter despite the difference in weight on the bar.

The basic requirements for a well-executed "conventional" deadlift are as follows.

Stance: Assume a stance that approximates the position you would take in order to perform a vertical leap. This will vary from individual to individual, but for most will roughly involve placing the feet under the hips as shown below.

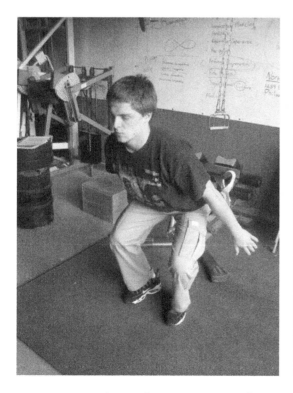 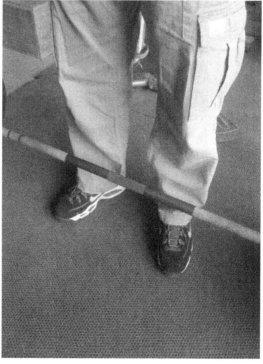

Assuming a stance as if you were to perform a vertical leap.

Grip: Take a grip on the bar that has your arms hanging perpendicular to the ground when viewed from the front. It is perfectly appropriate to use an "alternate" grip, meaning that one handed is facing out and one is facing in. Many argue that this negates the grip training effect of the deadlift, to which I say that the deadlift is primarily used to strengthen the musculature of the back, hamstrings, and glutes, all of which are significantly stronger than the grip, and suffer a decreased training effect when the loads are dictated by the strength of the weakest link in the chain. The same goes for the "hook" grip, which is acceptable if there is an interest in pursuing the sport of Olympic Weightlifting.

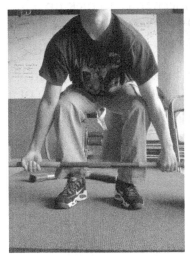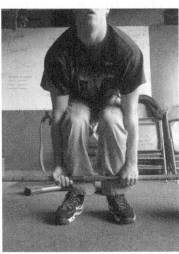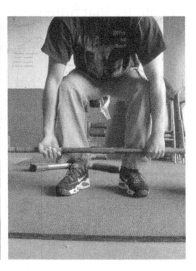

Deadlift Grip widths from left to right: too wide, too narrow, just right

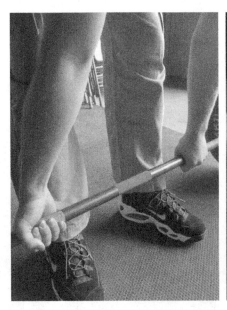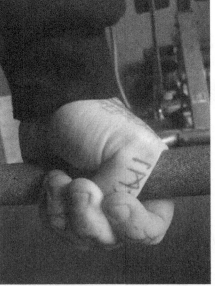

Left to Right: The Alternate Grip, The Hook Grip

Straps are also acceptable to use in training the deadlift, and many other lifts covered in this book. I am of the opinion that straps fall into the same category as a belt in terms of their appropriateness in a strength-training program. Remember, our desired outcome is building strength, and therefore our decisions about training need to be congruent with that outcome, not influenced or dictated by the opinions of others who have little invested in our actual performance and satisfaction.

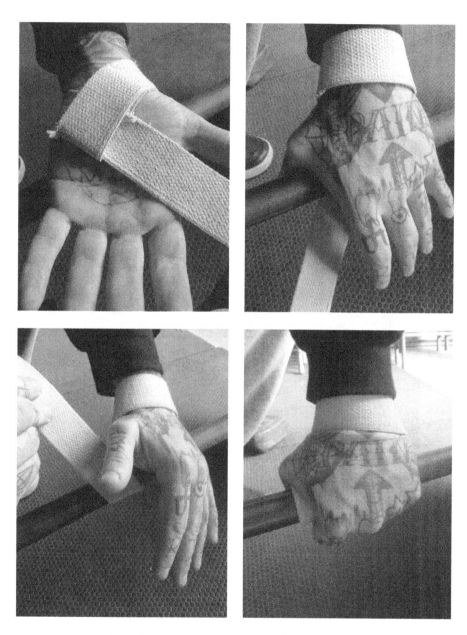

Detail on strap use: Crank them up tight

Position: Once the stance is assumed, and the grip is taken, the lifter then pushes out the chest, and drops the butt in order to place a nice arch in the back. The knees are pushed out a bit more in order to facilitate a bit of additional tightness. The butt will be positioned somewhere between the shoulders and the knees when viewed from the side. Where exactly the butt sits will depend on the build of the lifter.

For instance, a lifter with a back that is short relative to their femurs will have a back position that is more horizontal in appearance than one who is proportioned the opposite way (short femurs, long back). For this reason, deciding on an arbitrary "correct" angle for the back in the deadlift is impossible.

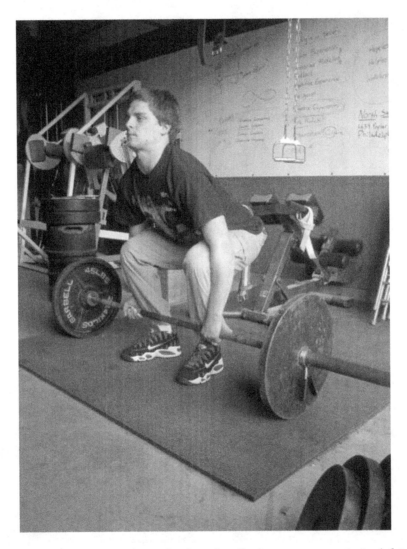

A good Deadlift start position minus the fact that Joe's arms are not straightened out yet.

Execution: Once the proper position is assumed, the last step before the bar breaks the floor happens in two parts.

1. The lifter takes all of the "slack" out of the bar, creating as much tightness as possible.
2. The lifter pushes his or her butt to the rear until they experience the sensation that they are going to lose their balance and fall over.

As soon as the lifter experiences that sensation, the bar is squeezed off of the ground and lifted until the hips and knees are extended and the lifter is standing upright. This completes the deadlift.

Returning the bar to the ground involves reversing the process "loosely", resisting gravity only enough to slow the bars descent and keep it from free-falling to the floor, creating a loud, douchey crash.

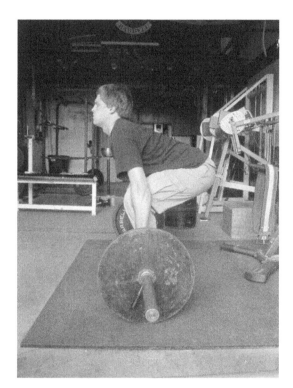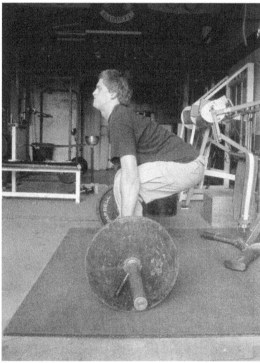

The last step before the bar breaks the floor. Note the butt shifting back towards the wall. Once the lifter gets the sensation that they are about to lose their balance, the bar is squeezed off of the floor.

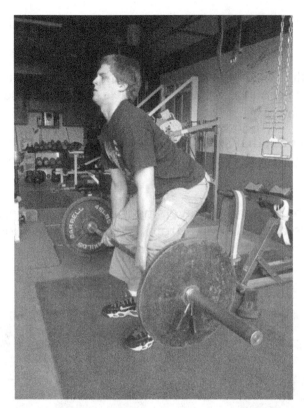

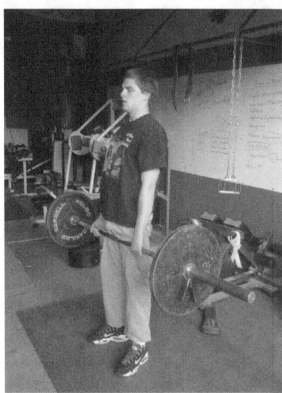

The Deadlift in execution

The Sumo Deadlift

The Sumo Deadlift is, in my opinion, the more natural of the two major deadlift movements. I feel that it more closely resembles how human beings pick objects up off of the ground than the conventional deadlift. It is for this reason that I have found it simpler to teach a lifter to perform correctly than the conventional pull.

Combine this observation with the idea that it is entirely possible to develop as much (if not more in some cases) strength and muscle using the sumo deadlift as the primary pulling movement, and one can ascertain my logic in often recommending the sumo variation as the big pull in a strength-training program.

In addition to being at least as effective as the conventional at building strength, our number one priority, the sumo deadlift is also legal in Powerlifting competitions for those who choose to compete in the sport. Another benefit of the movement, particularly for females who were not blessed with as ample of an ass as they would like is the profound ability for the sumo deadlift to promote significant development in the glutes.

Think of the sumo deadlift vs. the conventional deadlift less like a Phillips vs. a slotted screwdriver, and more like a Stanley Phillips screwdriver vs. a Craftsman Phillips screwdriver. Basically they are brother lifts that can accomplish the same task. Make your selection based on which you feel more comfortable with, or alternate the methods in your training. In either case you will reap the rewards of picking heavy weights up from the ground.

Performing the sumo deadlift is very simple, and involves performing the same steps as the conventional deadlift with one major difference.

Stance: The sumo deadlift uses a wider stance than the conventional deadlift, hence its name (the position looks similar to the position a sumo wrestler assumes before the match). It is common to see a very exaggeratedly wide stance used, particularly with powerlifters who are interested mainly in shortening the distance of the pull in order to let them move a few more pounds in competition. I do not advocate that style of stance for strength training. A correct sumo stance in my book has the shins perpendicular with the ground. The legs need to push into the ground as in the squat, and therefore should be in a position that maximizes their ability to do so.

Think of the lower legs as the legs of an "H" and not of an "M".

A decent rule for determining the correct stance width is to have the lifter stand in their squat stance. The two are remarkably similar in most cases.

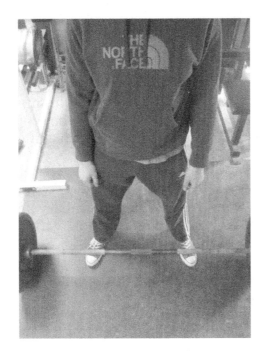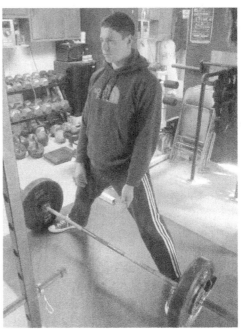

On the left, Drago takes his squat stance at the bar. On the right he demonstrates a stance that is much too wide.

Grip: Once the stance taken, the hands come down to the bar. Here we use the same rule as the conventional deadlift in that we want the arms to hang vertically, perpendicular to the bar and the floor. Again, it is appropriate to use an alternate grip or straps if desired.

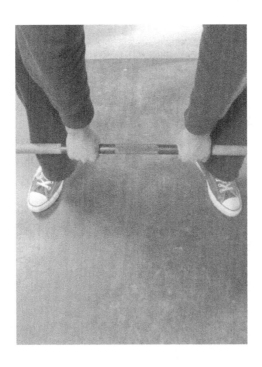

Position: The process for assuming the correct sumo deadlift can be summed to most by simply instructing them to "stand like a gorilla". By this I mean stand with the chest out and your butt low. Most everyone can produce a visual of this on command (unless they have never seen a gorilla).

The most significant piece of the position step is making sure that the chest is pushed out hard, and the lower back is "set" read: arched.

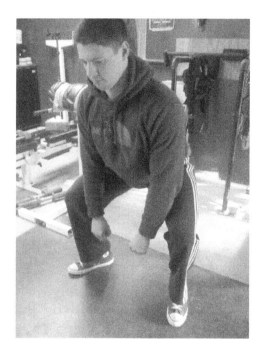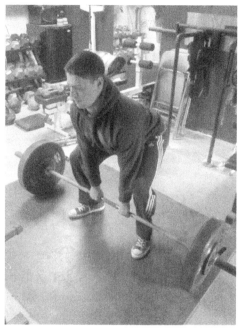

Drago stands "like a gorilla" in the photo to the left; note the similarity between the gorilla stance and the correct Sumo Deadlift start position.

Execution: As in the conventional deadlift, there are two steps to the last portion of the sumo deadlift prior to the bar leaving contact with the floor.

1. The lifter takes all of the "slack" out of the bar, creating as much tightness as possible.
2. The lifter pushes his or her butt to the rear until they experience the sensation that they are going to lose their balance and fall over.

As soon as the lifter experiences that sensation, the bar is squeezed off of the ground and lifted until the hips and knees are extended and the lifter is standing upright. This completes the sumo deadlift.

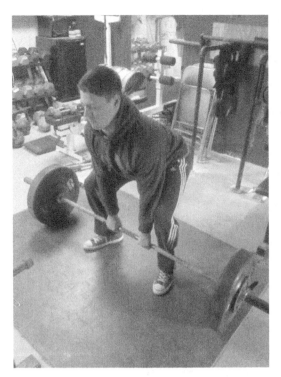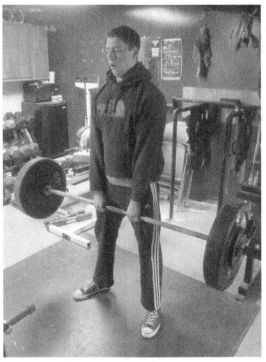

The Sumo Deadlift

Again, returning the bar to the ground involves reversing the process "loosely", resisting gravity only enough to slow the bars descent and keep it from free-falling to the floor, creating a loud, douchey crash. In case you haven't picked up on it yet, douchey crashes are not a good thing in my book.

The Rack Pull

I have a serious love for the rack pull. It has a very powerful feeling to it, and builds size and strength as well as any other lift in the arsenal. I perform and teach the rack pull different than many in that I set the pins in the rack so that bar is positioned slightly above the knee, on the thigh.

Performance of the rack pull is extremely simple. In order to do it correctly, place your hands on the bar using an alternate grip, or even better, straps, and apply good deadlift mechanics. By this I mean assume the stance you would use for a conventional deadlift, push out your chest, and take all of the "slack" out.

Squeeze the bar like hell, and keeping the chest pushed out, shove the feet into the floor. There is little coaching necessary for this one, just strength and a high pain tolerance for higher rep sets.

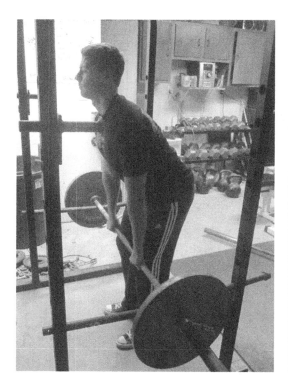 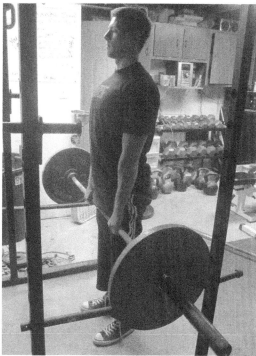

The Bench Press

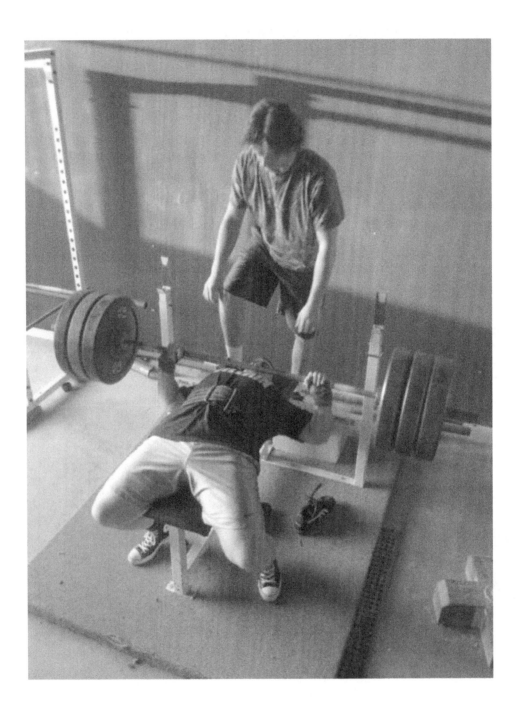

This is perhaps the most widely used barbell exercise in the world. As with the other lifts, I feel that people make teaching the bench press what I call "proprietarily complex" meaning that there is money to be made in over-complicating the safe performance of the lift. There are some things to account for in performing a bench press safely, but one needs to remember that this lift is performed everyday in gyms all of the world by people who have received no formal coaching on the movement.

The biggest issue that I have observed with flat benching, particularly when it is performed to the exclusion of any other bench press movements, is the risk of shoulder injury. The correlation between flat benching and bad shoulders has long steered bodybuilders towards the incline and decline variations of the lift where the risk is considerably reduced. Many will tell you that this is because the bodybuilders do not understand proper bench mechanics, and that is probably true to a degree, but the fact is that many powerlifters suffer shoulder injuries in training and competition on the flat bench as well.

The flat bench need not be avoided as a default, but it is critical to understand a few basic components of a well-executed bench press.

Tightness is key with the bench press. Nothing should be "slacked", the upper back should be firmly pressed into the bench, the lower back slightly arched, and the feet pressed firmly into the floor. It is acceptable to push the balls of the feet into the ground and have your heels up as in a "feet under" style, as well as having your feet flat as in a "feet forward" style.

The shoulders should be tucked behind you. Imagine trying to touch your shoulder blades together on the bench, or if you are versed in anatomy, picture the two scapulae laying flat on the surface of the bench with little space in between them. This changes the movement in terms of how it affects the shoulder, and decreases significantly the risk of injury.

I'll share with you a method I have long used for assuming a correct bench press position and executing a proper bench press.

Lay on the bench with your head hanging over the end. Grip the bar with the desired grip. Grip width will vary, but should result with the forearms being perpendicular with the ground when at the bottom of the movement.

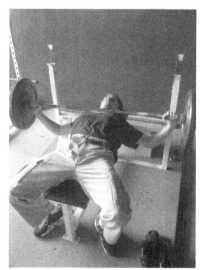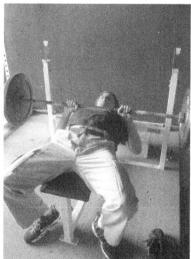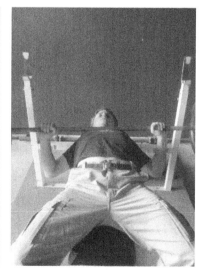

Left to Right: Too wide, too narrow, just right. Note the forearms are perpendicular to the floor when the bar is at the chest.

Plant your feet firmly in the ground. Use the bar to pull yourself down on the bench so that your nose is under the bar in the rack without moving the feet. Done correctly, this will create an arch in the low back, keep your butt on the bench, and create a great deal of tightness in the rest of the body.

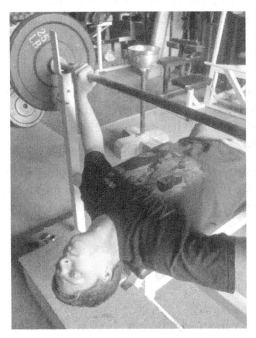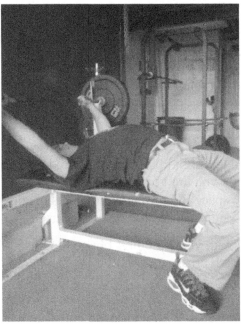

Joe begins by laying on the bench with his head hanging off. His feet are planted firmly and he uses the bar to pull himself down the bench, creating an arch in his lower back.

Once you're there, tuck the shoulders behind you, pushing the chest up towards the sky.

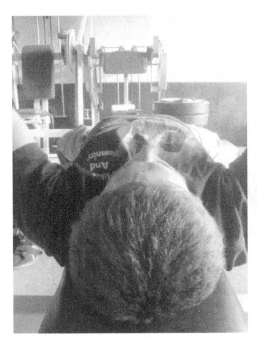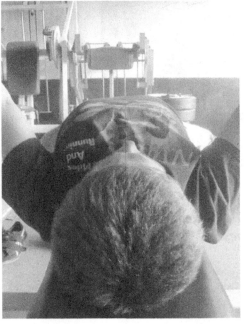

Joe pulls his shoulders together underneath him and pushes his chest to the sky.

After those simple steps are followed to assume the correct position, have a spotter help you take the bar from the rack and lower it to the chest, touching it slightly, then press the bar to lockout, keeping the shoulders tucked behind you. Breathe only at the top of the movement, as the rule states; never breathe while a bar is moving.

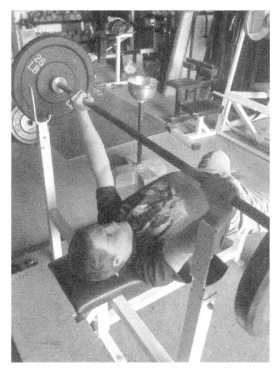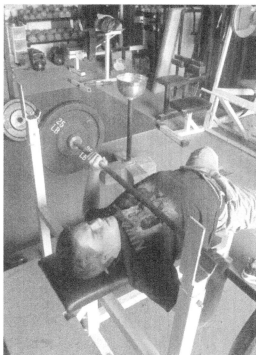

Joe lowers the bar to his chest, touching it gently, before returning the bar to lockout.

There is much more that has been, and can be written on the subject of the bench press. What you have now is enough technique to be dangerous as they say. Applying the ideas presented here will be a solid enough foundation for you to develop a tremendous amount of strength and muscle.

The Press

The press and the deadlift are arguably the simplest barbell lifts in theory. The idea of putting things over one's head I imagine has existed since people started picking things up. Few lifts produce the strength and muscular development benefits that the press is capable of when performed correctly.

Performing the press is simple. The first step is determining the proper grip. A correct pressing grip will have the forearms oriented perpendicular to both the ground and the bar when viewed from the front. For many males, this will involve placing the index fingers on the line where the smooth portion of the bar meets the knurling. It is critical that the wrists stay locked throughout the movement. The wrists should not be extended at all during any portion of the lift.

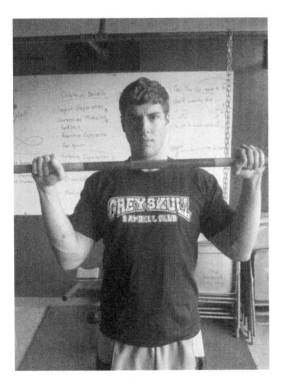 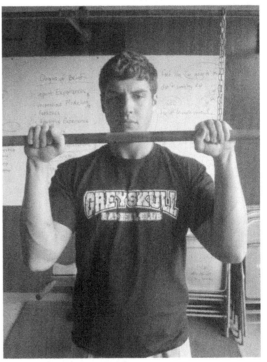

The first photo shows Devin taking a grip that is too wide. The second shows a grip that has the forearms perpendicular to both the bar, and the floor. This is a recurring theme in my teaching of the barbell lifts.

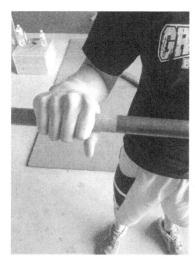 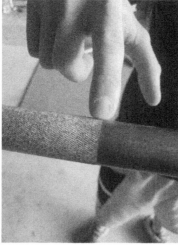 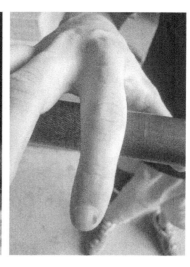

Devin illustrates a grip that is too wide in the rack. In the second photo he is indicating the point where the knurling of the bar meets the smooth; this is where most will place their index fingers to have correct grip spacing. Note: For reference, Devin is six foot four inches tall. If you are five foot eight inches, there is no possible way that your grip needs to be wider than his.

The chest should be flexed hard, which will in turn contract the lats and "tighten the armpits" creating a shelf that the triceps will rest on at the beginning, and bounce off of on the latter reps. Resting the triceps on this shelf will place the elbows in front of the body, but still pointed towards the ground. There is no need for the bar to touch the chest or collarbone area, as some will have you believe. One of the most common faults that I correct in lifters in the press is the resultant loss of tightness due to the perceived belief that it is necessary for the bar to rest on the front of the shoulders or the chest.

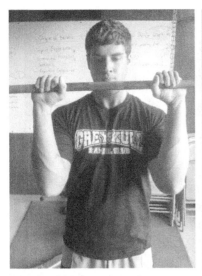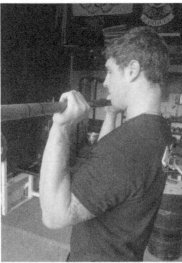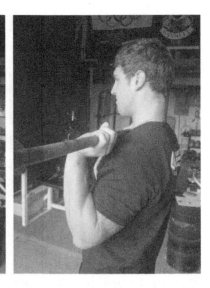

Flexing the chest to create the lat shelf. In the second photo, Devin is maintaining a straight wrist and allowing the bar to sit where it wants to, several inches off of his chest. Note the position of the elbow in the third picture when Devin relaxes the wrists in order to allow the bar to touch the chest. The erroneous belief that the bar needs to touch the body leads to a loosening of the entire supportive platform.

The stance should be the same as the squat, a bit wider than most tend to stand naturally when attempting the movement.

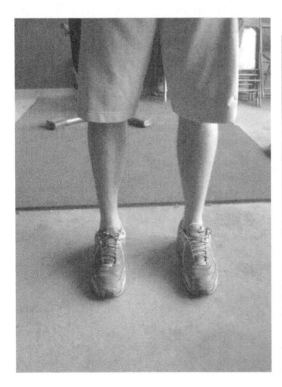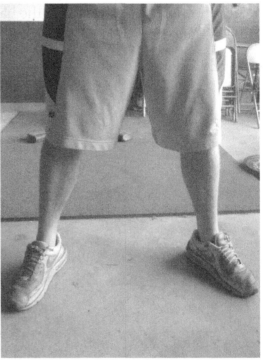

In the left photo Devin demonstrates a stance that is too narrow. In the photo on the right he takes his squat stance, the appropriate stance for the Press.

The first rep is performed by taking a giant breath in and holding it in before shoving the bar to lockout over the head. Once the bar is locked out, the breath is released slightly, a new breath is taken and the bar is lowered quickly but under control in order to "bounce" off of the shelf created by the lats for the next rep. To make this effect more pronounced, I instruct lifters to imagine performing a "pec-dec flye" throughout the movement, both on the way up, and the way down. This kinesthetic modeling creates the tightness needed to effectively use the upper body musculature synergistically, and move the weight efficiently.

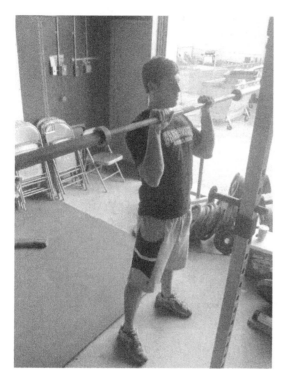 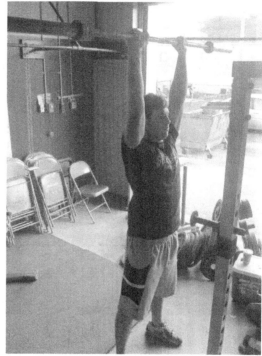

The Press

A pause is appropriate if deemed necessary at the top of the movement, but never at the bottom. After the first rep is performed, all subsequent reps begin at the top (think squat instead of deadlift). As always, no breathing occurs while the bar is in motion.

The Incline Bench Press

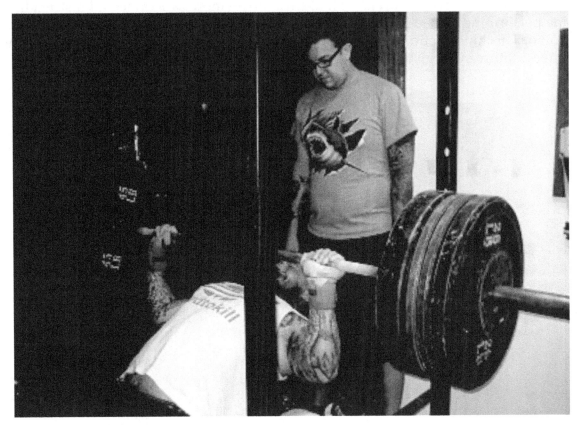

The author training the Incline Bench Press

The incline bench press has been used in the bodybuilding community for decades. Its ability for building strength and muscle is legendary. Many regard it as an inferior lift to the flat bench press, though I thoroughly disagree. It is true that less weight is used in the incline version than the flat in almost every case, but in terms of strength development, weight is not the only variable that matters.

Interestingly enough, in discussion with Bill Starr, strength legend, and author of "The Strongest Shall Survive", he told me that he largely preferred the incline to the flat bench, and only included the latter in his book because at the time most football programs did not yet have access to incline benches. He said that everyone had benches, even if they were the locker room variety, and could therefore perform the flat bench. He was speaking to his audience.

Bodybuilders prefer the incline (and decline) bench press to the flat due to the dramatic reduction in shoulder injuries seen with the former methods.

The flat bench is certainly an effective lift, but it is by no means the only bench press version worth mentioning in this book, or applying in your strength-training program.

The incline bench requires significantly less "technique" than the flat bench. Tucking the shoulders behind you is ideal in the movement still, but far from necessary. Most all who attempt the incline bench press will perform what I would consider an effective repetition on their first try.

Many incline benches are set at a fixed angle. If selecting one of these from a variety, I prefer a shallow incline to a steeper incline. If you are using an adjustable bench, opt for something a step or two above flat. Forty-five degrees is a bit steep for me, but honestly, I still prefer it to the flat bench.

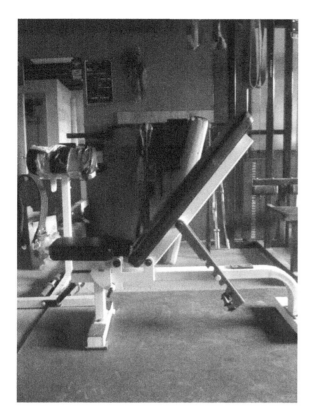 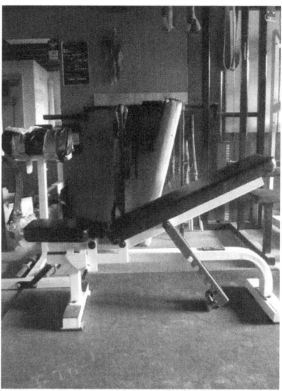

An adjustable Incline Bench. The left photo shows an incline that is too steep for my liking. The right photo is just right.

The Close Grip Bench Press

The close-grip is another go-to favorite of mine for myself and others. The lift is much easier on the shoulders than the standard bench press, and therefore is a favorite amongst older lifters, athletes, and anyone else whose shoulders are of great importance.

The training effect of the close-grip is very similar to that of the flat bench press (the decline and incline versions can also be performed with a close grip). The chest, shoulders, and triceps are all heavily involved in the movement as they are in the standard bench, despite the classification that many have of the close grip as a tricep exercise exclusively.

There are two basic variations to the close grip bench press. There is the more "powerlifting" friendly version which involves having the upper arms remain in contact and "rub" the torso throughout the lift (a movement which resembles the action of a shirted bench press), and the "bodybuilding" version which involves letting the elbows "do what they want" and drift out a bit. Both styles work well, though I am more of a fan of the "bodybuilding" style, even for those for whom strength is number one priority.

Spacing of the hands is simple in the close grip. The grip should be virtually identical to the grip used for the press. Oh, and like the other pressing movements, don't be an ass, put your thumb around the bar.

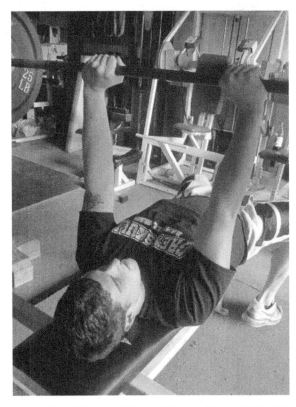 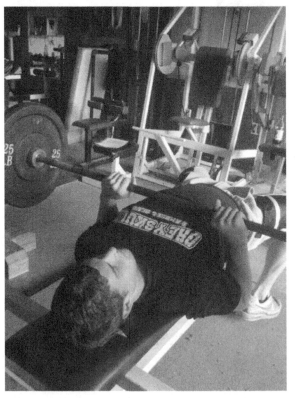

The "Powerlifting" Style Close-Grip Bench Press; elbows in tight the whole time.

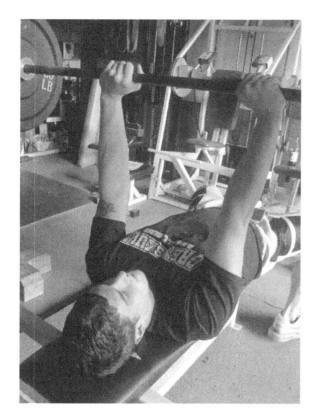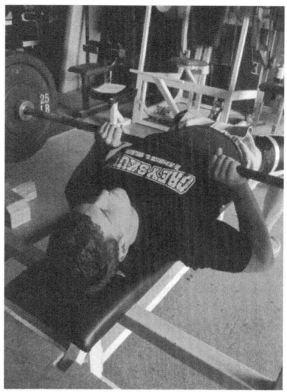

The "Bodybuilding" style Close-Grip Bench Press; Elbows do what they want.

The Decline Bench Press

The decline bench press is perhaps my favorite upper body movement with the exception of the press. The ability to move a significant amount of weight in a surprisingly natural feeling motion gives great kinesthetic feedback throughout the movement. If you are unfamiliar with the lift it will be difficult to understand what I am saying, but those who have moved big loads on a decline bench can certainly relate.

Dorian Yates regards the decline bench as the best exercise for developing the pectorals due to it most closely resembling the movement that the pecs are responsible for naturally. He used the lift extensively in developing his gargantuan chest and upper body, and I followed suit with many others and myself in my training career.

If you have access to a decline bench press and you've never used it, you're definitely shitting the bed.

As with the other bench press movements (arguably more so with the decline) it is critical to have a spotter to help in the event that you cannot move the bar. An alternative to this is using (dare I say it) a Smith Machine. Don't ask me why these things are so hated. Lots of really big, really strong people disagree that leprosy is a result of using them.

The Front Squat

The front squat is a very effective tool for building strength, and muscle, particularly in the quads and glutes. The lift has long been a staple in Olympic Weightlifting programs, its obvious application in that instance being the development of the specific strength necessary to stand up with a heavy clean before the clean and press. It has also been used extensively in the bodybuilding community for decades as a quad-blasting squat variant.

No matter the variation of the front squat, the results are always solid.

The "Olympic" front squat, as we will call it, is performed by holding the barbell in the "rack" position of the clean and then performing a squat.

The bodybuilding style front squat is performed by crossing the arms in front of the body as shown below, elbows out, hands in fists touching opposite shoulders. This creates a shelf to rest the bar on. The bodybuilding style is simpler to perform correctly, though it requires that the bar be taken out of a rack or off of a stand. The Olympic style does not require a rack, as the bar can be cleaned into place.

Both styles have their applications. I feel no obligation to recommend the Olympic style front squat to anyone other than those interested in competing in the sport. In terms of building strength and muscle, the bodybuilding variation will certainly get the job done.

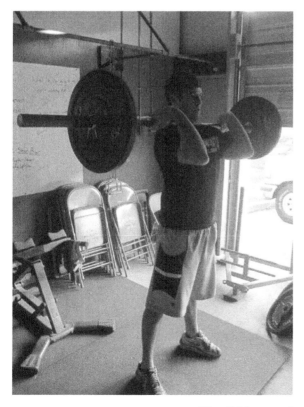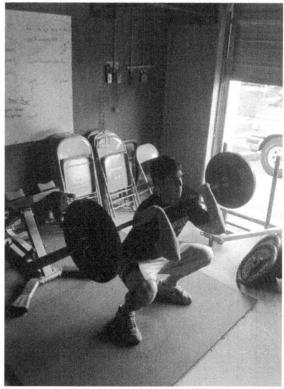

The "Olympic" style Front Squat

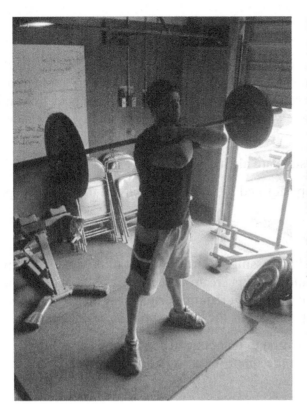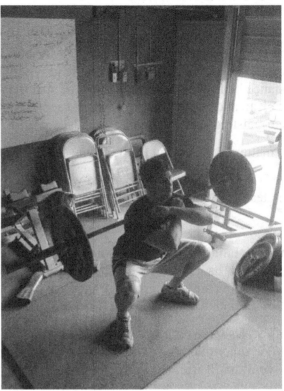

The "Bodybuilding" style Front Squat

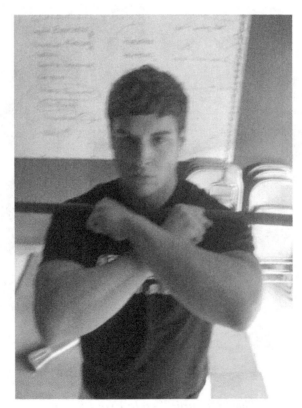

Detail on Bar Position; Keep those elbows out!

The Deficit Deadlift

The deficit is an extremely effective tool for developing strength from the floor. I use the lift extensively with individuals who have gotten stuck on the conventional or sumo deadlift in terms of making forward progress. As I address in some of my other products, the effectiveness of this lift in that application has less to do with a particular characteristic of the lift, and more to do with the effect of perceived change of stimulus in the lifter's brain, particularly if they are the of the traditional "program shopper" ilk.

In addition to using the lift to help many get "unstuck", I have used the lift many times as a contrast prior to having a lifter attempt a personal record deadlift from the floor. Commonly I have observed a lifter pull a heavy single or double from a deficit, after which I remove the deficit, add weight, and have the lifter pull from the floor. This has resulted in a personal record deadlift for many of my trainees over the years.

The execution of the deficit deadlift is simple. It follows the same steps as the conventional deadlift outlined before. The only major difference in the position is that the hips will be much higher than in the pull from the floor.

The only additional equipment that is required is a platform of some sort for the lifter to stand on that is higher than the floor. Three and a half inches has long been the magic number at Greyskull. There is no scientific reason for this figure, it is simply the height of one our thirty-five pound rubber bumper plates, which are rarely used and therefore available for standing on, plus a piece of half-inch plywood.

The lift can be performed from lesser heights; I am only sharing the three and a half inch idea for some reference.

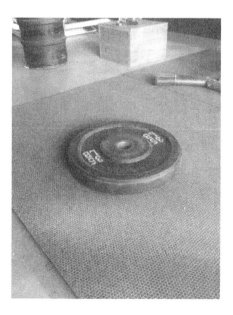

The deficit platform; in this case a rarely used thirty-five pound bumper plate.

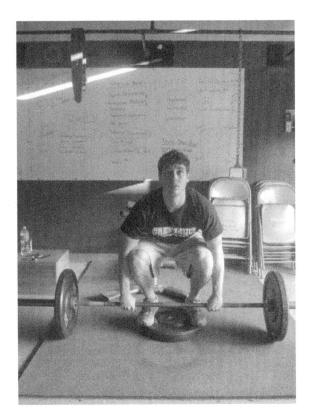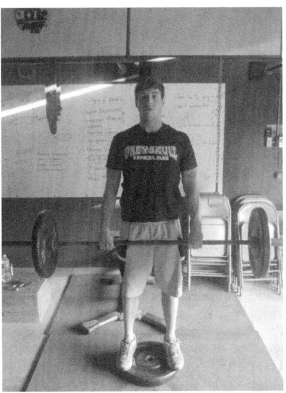

The Deficit Deadlift

The Trap Bar Deadlift

The trap bar is a great general-purpose type tool to have around the gym. There are many uses for the thing. Personally I use the trap bar more for conditioning purposes, normally as a farmers walk implement in conjunction with a dragging sled, but it is also a more than acceptable bar to use for deadlifting.

The trap bar deadlift is extremely similar to the conventional deadlift in terms of setup. There is no real need to elaborate on this. The largest difference in setup is the grip width, which is dictated by the spacing of the handles on the bar anyway.

If you have access to a trap bar, it is perfectly acceptable to use it as part of this program.

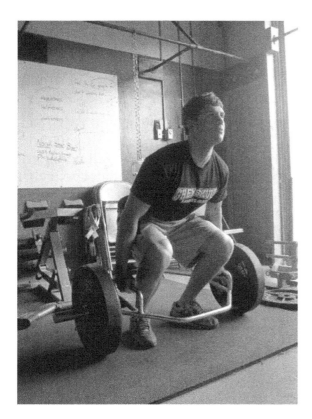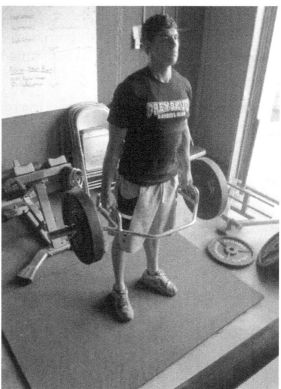

The Trap Bar Deadlift

The Power Snatch

The Olympic lifts have long been noted for their athletic benefits in terms of developing explosive power. There certainly is a place for the snatch and or clean and jerk in a well-designed strength-training program.

I am of the opinion that the "power" versions of the lifts, where the lifter does not drop into a squat to catch the weight, work very well for this purpose. I am biased towards the power snatch when designing programs for others for two reasons; its relative simplicity when compared to the power clean, and its usability by a more diverse population. I have worked with many people, male and female, who were unable to perform a solid "rack" position without considerable practice and/or stretching. If the lifter desires to compete in the sport of Olympic Weightlifting, then developing the rack position is a fact of life. If not however, there is no real need to do so in order to reap the benefits of the lifts.

Performing a power snatch is simpler than it may appear. Again, there are many who can and will go on for hours about the proper execution of the power snatch. I am not one of those people. It's a good idea to find an Olympic Weightlifting coach in your area to work on the finer points of the lifts with if you plan on pursuing the sport. If not, this technique primer will do the trick.

Begin by determining your snatch grip. This is accomplished by holding an empty barbell at roughly waist height with a wide grip as shown. Try lifting one of your knees. If you cannot lift your knee up in front of you without the barbell interfering, move your grip out wider until the bar sits in the crease of the hip when the knee is raised. Virtually no one will instinctively grip the bar too wide, but if you find that you feel exaggeratedly wide, or the bar is nowhere near your hip crease, you may need to narrow your grip a bit.

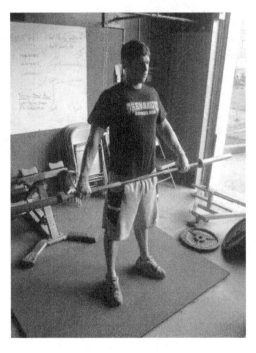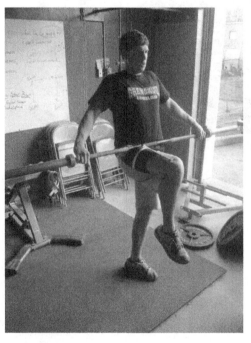

Determining the correct grip spacing

Make note of the position of your hands on the bar, this will be your snatch grip.
Stand at the barbell using a conventional deadlift stance, turning your toes out just slightly more than usual. Grip the bar using the snatch grip, and push the chest out hard, arching the back.

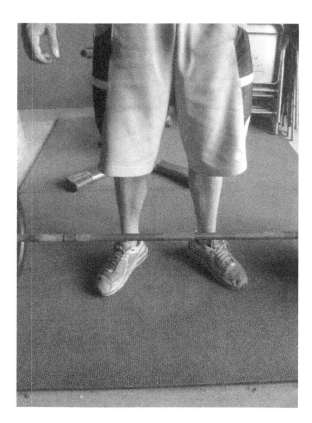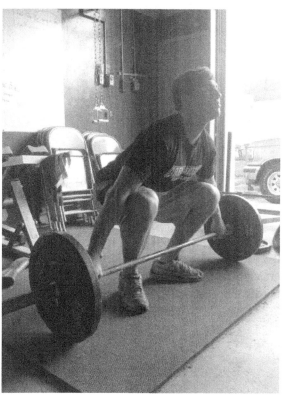

The start position for the Power Snatch: Note the toes are slightly more turned out that with the Deadlift.

Begin the lift by squeezing the bar from the floor. When the bar reaches about the middle of your thigh, jump and put the bar up over your head. When done correctly, the bar should hit your belly on the way up, and should not have any sort of arc to its trajectory. Straight up. It may help to imagine performing the lift in front of a wall or in a smith machine to illustrate the correct bar path.

Continued on next page…

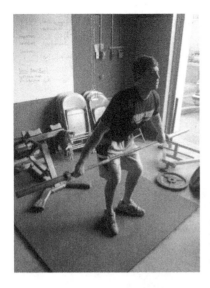 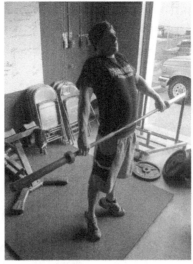 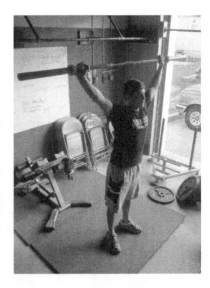

The Power Snatch: the jump occurs when the bar hits the mid-thigh.

To bring the bar down, lower it in a controlled manner, and replace it on the floor. Dropping the bar is en vogue, but still lame. Remember that guys lowered bars with three or four times the weight you are using fifty years ago before rubber bumper plates became the fashion.

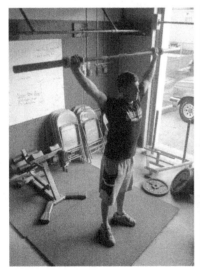 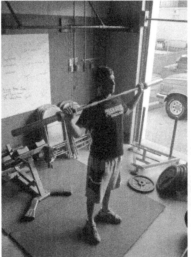 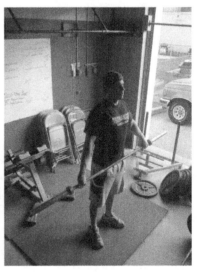

Lowering the bar

The Weighted Chin-up

These are invaluable as a builder of upper back, upper arm, and forearm musculature, as well as being a hell of a tool for developing savage overall upper body strength. I greatly prefer and advocate the use of the chin-up (palms facing you) over the pull-up (palms facing away) for several reasons. The most important (to me) reason for the use of the chin-up over the pull-up is that often grip is the limiting factor in the pull-up. The pull-up is a terrific exercise as well, but most will attest that they can perform at least a few more chins than they can pull-ups. The pull-up is the more challenging exercise simply because less muscle is operating in a mechanically advantageous manner. This is one of those bizarre instances where the belief exists for many that the 'harder' version must be better. My belief is whatever movement allows you to use the most weight for the most repetitions will invariably get you the strongest and consequently develop the most muscle mass.

Rest assured that if you train chins and weighted chins hard; you will never be a slouch at performing pull-ups. They will always trail behind in number, but will always be there just a few steps behind when you need them (this is important to note, considering I advocate the use of chin-ups for building strength in military personnel who actually test on the pull-up).

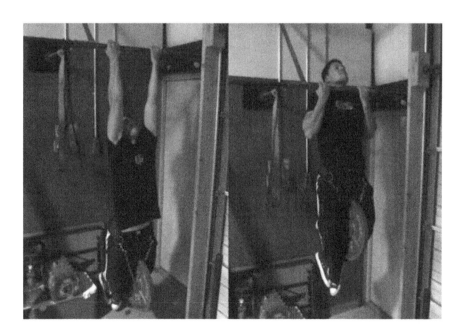

To perform the weighted chin, don a weight belt and hang from a bar with your palms facing towards you as shown. Make it a dead hang, meaning that the elbows are not bent at all. From there pull up until your throat comes in contact with the bar.

In more cases than not I will have the trainee perform the weighted chins on the same day(s) of the week that they press. This means that every second workout the trainee is performing the weighted chin.

The movement will be done for two working sets in the six to eight rep range. This means that the trainee will strive to reach failure (when they cannot complete another repetition; easy to find with this exercise) between six and eight repetitions.

They will then take a short rest, the duration of which is determined by how they are feeling and when they are ready to have at it again (shouldn't exceed five minutes, however), and knock out another set with the intention of reaching failure somewhere between six and eight reps again.

There are many ways to improve with rep range-style training. This idea is one of the core principles of the 'Powerbuilding' methods we use here for more advanced, hypertrophy-seeking individuals (there will be much more written about these methods in later works). One can use the same weight for both sets, in which case they will likely not repeat the same number of reps on the second set, or reduce the weight used on the belt for the second set. Either is fine, so long as the trainee is making some measure of improvement in either weight used or reps completed from workout to workout (barring the occasional and understandable exception). Below are some examples:

Workout 1: 10 lbs x 6 reps on first set, 7.5 lbs x 7 reps on second set. (Trainee has made the desired rep range on both sets so he is cleared to either increase the weight used on one or both sets, or keep the weight the same and try to get deeper into the rep range).

Workout 2: 10 lbs x 7 reps on first set, 10 lbs x 6 reps on second set. (Here the trainee kept the weight the same and beat his reps from the first set of the last workout. After the first set, he opted to maintain the same load on the belt and go for it since the first set felt pretty good. He made fewer reps than he did on the first set, but it is still an improvement over his second set effort on the previous workout).

Workout 3: 12.5 lbs x 6 reps on first set, 7.5 lbs x 7 reps on second set. (Here the trainee pushed the weight up on the first set and barely managed to get six reps. He did it though, and made the rep range. Since he was smoked from the effort however, he backed off the weight for the second effort. He got seven reps with the same weight he got seven with on workout one, but it is still a victory since he beat his weight record for six reps on the first set. Technically the second set is still an improvement since the first time he completed 7.5 lbs for seven reps he had not done 12.5 for six beforehand).

You can see from the above examples that progress is slow going on these, but small victories are the name of the game. Make your rep range, and add weight when you feel you can. You will also notice that the weights used on the belt were not terribly heavy. Many people, I believe, have a belief that weighted chin-ups are only for those who can hang a 45, or at least 25 lb, plate from the belt. This intimidation factor keeps many from taking on this excellent exercise. The weighted chin-up is to be trained linearly and loaded in small increments, just the same as any other weighted exercise.

The Yates Row

Made famous and named after Dorian Yates, this is without a doubt my favorite rowing movement. It admittedly is difficult for some to get the hang of, despite its simplicity and short range of motion, but learning to perform the lift correctly is well worth the effort.
The lift begins similar to a conventional deadlift in terms of stance. The grip is a bit narrower however; the hands should be inside of the hips as shown. The lifter picks the bar up from the ground, keeping the knees bent slightly, and assumes a back position that is near vertical. Some call this lift the seventy-degree row due to the angle of the back.

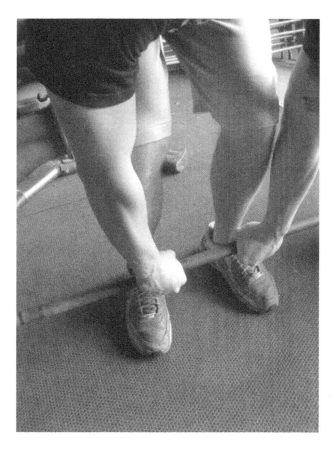

Position for the Yates row at the floor

The torso and lower-body remain motionless throughout the movement. The only portion of the body that moves is the arm. The elbows are driven back behind the body, bringing the bar into the bladder area. There is no pause with the Yates row, it is a power movement, and is used to move the heaviest weight possible without moving any other portion of the body.

Done correctly the Yates row will hammer the lats directly unlike any other movement.

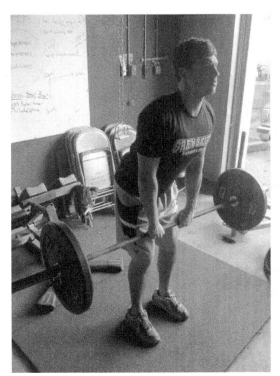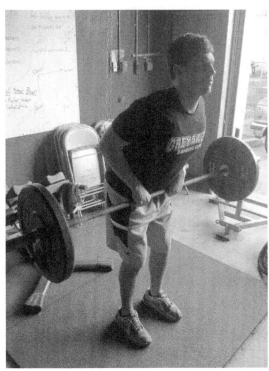

The Yates Row

The V-Handle Pulldown

I choose the v-handle for the Pulldown over the other able attachment options because of the resultant increase in range of motion, and the fact that it is possible to move greater loads than with a wide grip.

More weight plus more range of motion means more strength and muscle developed.
The lats are significantly stronger than the biceps and the forearms. As a result, opting for a version of the lift that involves those components more, and therefore designates them as the limiting factor in terms of performance of the lift, a lesser training effect is received.

When operating from an outcome-based perspective, it is critical that decisions are made in terms of what is going to produce the most significant result.

Performing the movement correctly is simple.

Sit upright in the seat with legs locked. Lock the lower back in extension, and push your chest out hard (it stays this way throughout). Reach until your shoulders are pulled up (as in a dead hang pull-up) and pull the handle down to your upper chest, driving with your elbows and thinking of your hands as hooks. Use straps preferably, but just say no to momentum.

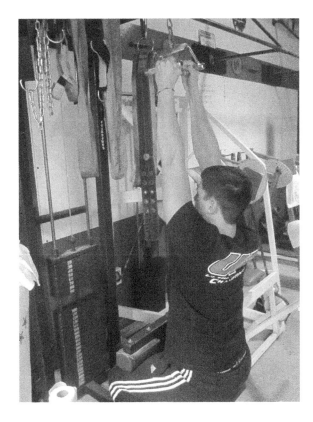
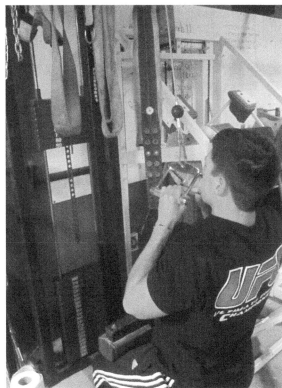

The Dumbbell Row

This one is simple and effective.

Despite its simplicity, many often perform this movement with horrible form. The movement is smooth from start to finish, not jerky and rapid nature as if you were starting a lawnmower. The weight hangs dead at the beginning of each rep and is then "rowed" back towards the hip (not up towards the pec line as you will see many do).

Tension is key in the rowing movements. Everything should be "squeezed" hard. A slight pause is appropriate at the top of the movement. The pause should not be long enough to require that candy weights be used on the movement, but enough to allow a hard contraction to take place. We're talking half a second here, tops.

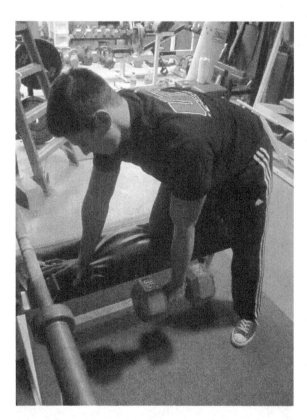
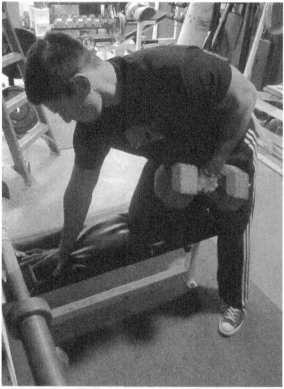

The Curl Variants

The curl has gotten such a bad rap in certain circles in recent years it is not even funny. There is some sort of strange belief that the curl is some sort of a weenie exercise that shouldn't be performed for fear that one may get all Liberace all of the sudden. This is ridiculous notion, and frankly the aversion that many have to the curl is beyond my comprehension.

Simply put, if you want an impressive, strong pair of arms, you should probably curl.

So am I saying that this is a vanity thing? Am I advocating the curl solely for cosmetic reasons? Well, yes and no.

There are those who like to make everything about 'functionality' as in 'where does the movement exist in nature?' This is silly to me because none of their highly touted movements occur in nature in the manner in which they train them (for those in the know on the CrossFit side of the fence, tell me when in the history of the world has anyone done anything that vaguely resembled "Fran" in any context). I say that humans perform elbow flexion while carrying loads in their hands in many situations. How do you carry grocery bags while you juggle for your keys?

But wait, damn it, you've got me talking like these weirdoes now. Let's cut the crap, we want big, strong arms and by God we're going to use the curl to get them. I like to have trainees curl on the days that they bench press. They fit into the program after the bench press is done for the day, and before the big lift is started. There will generally be two working sets done in the 10-15 rep range.

There are many incarnations of the curl, but we will be dealing with the three I most frequently use. I like to have the trainee rotate these three (or at least two of the three) from workout to workout, meaning that if we designated days that we bench press as "A" days that each "A" day will feature a different curl variant until he cycles back to the top of the order (in the case of using two variants, there is simply an "A1" and an "A2" workout).

Here are the favorites in no particular order.

The Standing EZ Curl Bar Curl

This is the most basic of the curl variants. I like the EZ curl bar because I find that it does not cause the wrist and forearm pain that a straight bar does in many, myself included. Any commercial gym will have plenty of these to use, and if you train at home, they are inexpensive and can always be had for a steal off of Craigslist.org if nothing else.

Some argue in book-nerd fashion that the EZ curl bar does not allow for full biceps involvement since the wrist is not supinated at the top as it is with a straight bar. I always say if I want to supinate the wrist, I can (and will) use dumbbells to accomplish the task in a more effective manner. The other common argument offered by some, which has always baffled me, is that the EZ curl bar curl involves too much contribution from the brachialis. A quick look at an anatomy chart will tell us that the brachialis is located in the upper arm, precisely the area we are trying to make bigger and stronger, so inviting it to the party certainly isn't a bad thing.

Simply put, for building big cannons, the EZ curl bar is the balls.

As a tip (the movement itself is best taught in person or on video, look for our free tutorial videos on strengthvillain.com for more detail) make everything as tight as possible when doing these. Flex your chest and lats hard throughout the whole movement. If you haven't learned how to consciously control these muscles, just imagine holding a pair of five-pound plates under your armpits while you perform the movement. Maintain this tightness at the top of the movement and lift your elbows up slightly at the end; you'll feel the whole unit get much tighter, and the bicep itself will feel as if it has no more potential to contract (which it won't). This small movement triggers the last little bit of contraction from the biceps proximal (closest to the body) function of contributing to the movement of the upper arm at the shoulder joint.

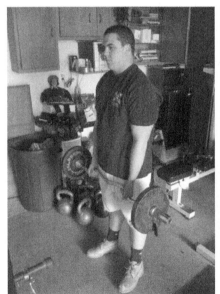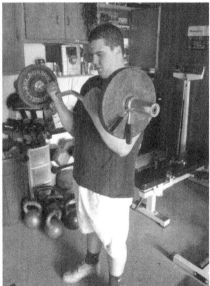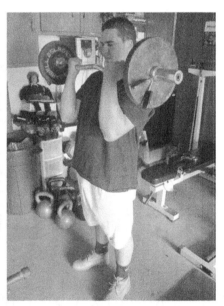

Zacl Demonstrating the EZ Curl Bar Curl. Note the squeeze and elevated elbows at the top of the movement.

The Seated Alternating Dumbbell Curl

It is important to note that when performing exercises that are trained with dumbbells, making small incremental increases in weight is not possible without the use of special equipment (magnetic add on weights; a solid investment for an aspiring bodybuilder). This is one reason for the greater gap in the rep range used for biceps movements (10-15) over movements which use involve more joints, use more muscle, and are trained with barbells. An increase of five pounds in one hand with a dumbbell is more significant than a 10 lb increase on a barbell. Combine that with the fact the curl uses a very small amount of muscle mass relative even to the press, and the five-pound increase in one hand becomes even more drastic. The trainee will have to start low in the rep range and endeavor to get well into the range, pushing close to if not all the way out to 15 reps before going up in weight. It is also likely, and often advisable, that the trainee will be well suited to use a lighter pair of dumbbells for the second set than for the first. The exception here would be a case where the lifter is close to maxing the rep range on the first set and is trailing it with a shorter set, still in the range, with the same dumbbells.

The photo below will show the correct grip on the dumbbell for curling.

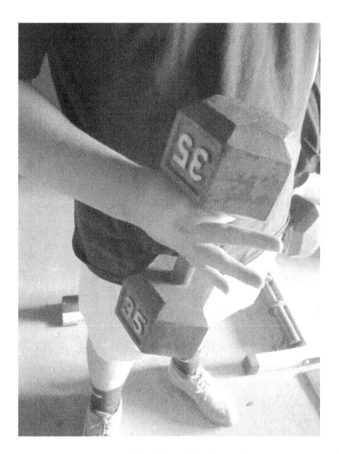

The correct placement of the Dumbbell in the hand for curling.

Holding the dumbbells in this manner makes the biceps work harder, against the longer lever arm, to supinate the wrist at the top of the movement. It adds a nasty twist to the movement and is great for spurring growth.

As with the standard EZ curl bar curl, keep everything flexed up tight throughout the movement. Imagine holding those five pounders under the armpits and *squeeze*!

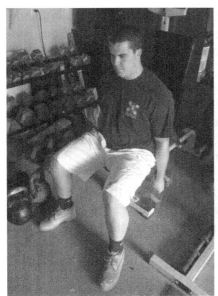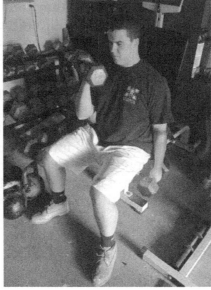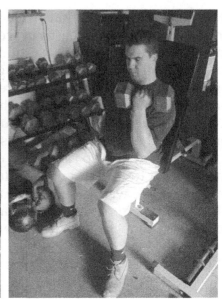

The Seated Alternating Dumbbell Curl

The EZ curl bar drag curl

This variation of the standard curl described above is one of my favorites. When done right, it provides one of the nastiest negatives you can create. This is better learned in person or with video (again, check out the tutorial vids at strengthvillain.com) but the photos below will give you the gist, experimentation will get you that 'a-ha' moment in time.

The concentric portion is the same as the normal curl.

On the negative portion, shoot your elbows back behind you, keeping your arms squeezed in tight to your sides, until the bar is touching the front of your torso (where it comes in contact with you will depend on individual limb segment lengths).

You then perform the negative by sliding the bar down the front of your body to the start position.

Ease into these, and remember that the movement is to be performed strict, and with a ton of tension throughout your entire body. Don't get sloppy on these, keep it strict Dorian style and get guns that you'll need permits for to carry in public (yes I really just said that).

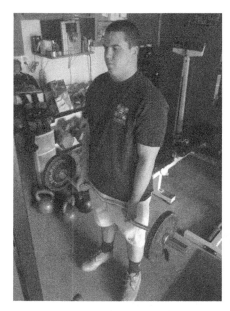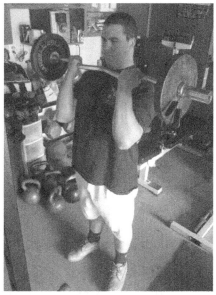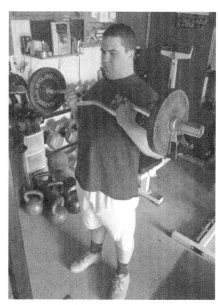

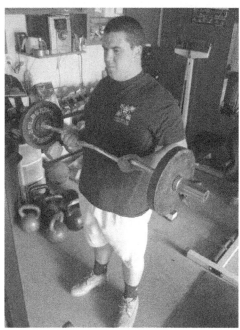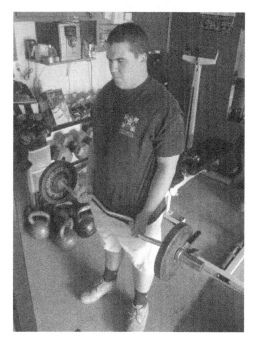

The EZ Curl Bar Drag Curl

The Neck Extension

This is one of the simplest of the weight room tasks, but is one of the most common things for people to ask me about. In the photos below Zack demonstrates how to do this awesome exercise correctly.

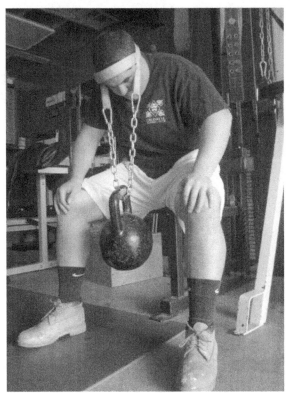
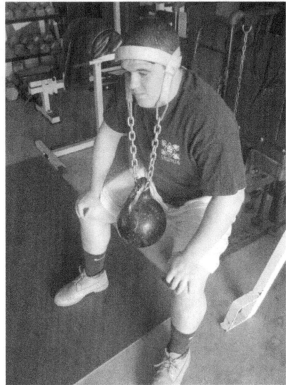

The Neck Extension using a Neck Harness

Start light with the neck harness. Pick a weight you can get for four sets of 25 reps, without straining too much. Trust me, it will be difficult to turn your head the next day even if you start out really light. The studliest of studs that are brand new to the harness should not try doing more than 25 lbs the first time.

Progress on the harness is possible in many ways and can be carried on more or less infinietly. Generally speaking we will start someone out with the 4 x 25 and increase the weights until we get to about 55 lbs (we typically won't exceed this weight, there is no need). At that point we will generally just increase the length of the sets. Zack (pictured) did four sets of 110 reps with a 55 lb kettlebell just a few days ago as I write this (added to show perspective on potential for progression, not to show how awesome Zack is, he doesn't need me to do that).

As long as you are using more weight or doing more reps, even if it is by a small margin on either or both, you are doing it right.

The harness is an awesome tool, and a Greyskull staple. A thick neck is a great insurance policy against injury, and makes you much harder to knock out, which is why it has been used for years by combat athletes like boxers and wrestlers, as well as by football and rugby players. Basically the cool kids do it so we will too.

It is not at all uncommon for us to see an inch and a half worth of growth on the neck measurement in six to eight weeks after adding them in.

Our people will typically do these every weight training session.

The G Row

I included this lift simply because I get a lot of questions about it. It works well as an overall "finisher" on the deadlift day or any day for that matter. It is a bit unconventional, but really works for developing the ability to maintain isometric contraction in the back throughout the squat, and for just general back development.

The lift sounds more complex than it is. Tightness, and smoothness of motion are the key points to remember on this one.

To perform a G row, Lie face down on a Glute Ham Developer holding a barbell. Perform a back extension, pausing at the top. Once at the top, row the barbell up to touch your chest and hold for a three count. After the three count, let the bar down first and then return to the bottom position.

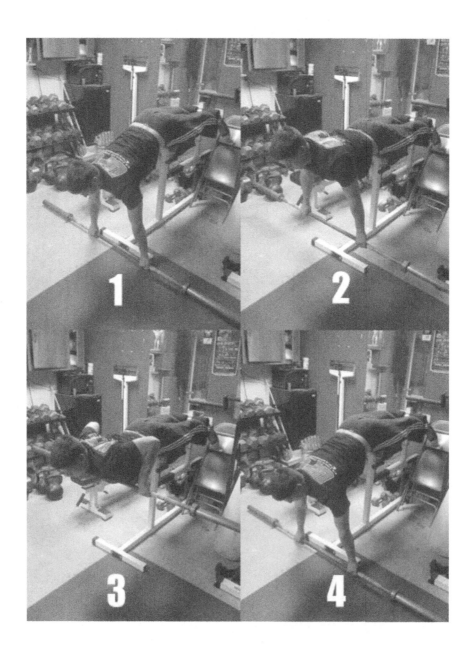

Conclusion

Well there you have it. That's the gist of the 'Greyskull LP'. Hopefully a lot of questions have been answered, some new information was digested, and you are ready to make some serious progress.

As I tell all of my clients, consistency is hands down the most important single variable in getting what you want out of your training. Determine what you want first, then reverse engineer the program that is most conducive to getting you there using the plug-ins noted to add to the base. Once you've got it all figured out, get after it and be consistent. I promise you will get where you want to go if you just keep pushing in that direction with intensity and focus on the prize.

As always I encourage you to contact me with any questions you may have.

I am also available for private consultations. My clients enjoy the rewards of learning how those who are tremendously successful in their chosen endeavors approach things mentally, and also enjoy custom-tailored programs designed for them with their individual desired outcome in mind.

I can be reached by email at john@villainintl.com

Or you can ask me questions in my Q and A section on my website strengthvillain.com

If you do make it over to strengthvillain.com I highly recommend starting a training log in the training logs section. This allows you to track your progress and have a layer of accountability, as well as providing me a look into what you have going on should you run into a snag and ask my assistance. I also do drop by people's logs at random, as do my knowledgeable moderators, so there are always eyes on you to provide help and support on your journey to whatever your goals may be.

Until next time, stay focused and keep producing the outcomes that you desire.

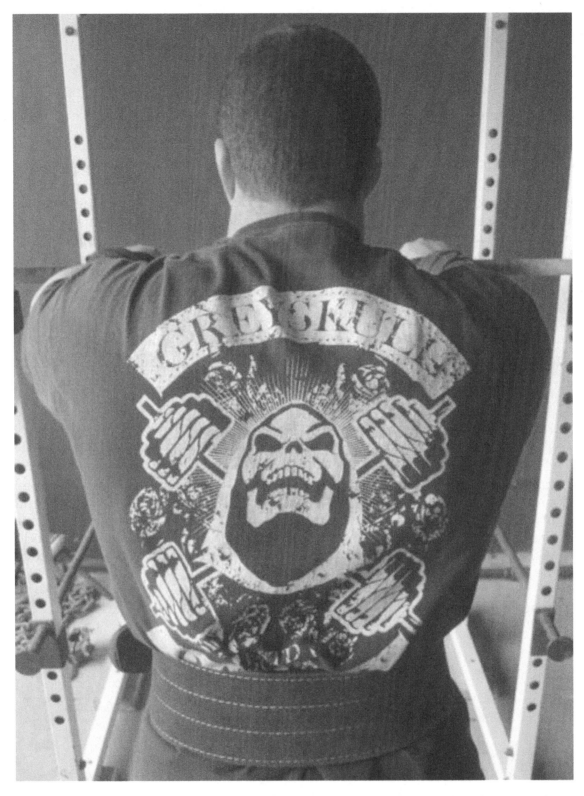

Special thanks to Zack, Joe, Devin, Drago, and Biggs, my models for this thing. Without their striking good looks, this would have just been a lot of bland text.

Made in the USA
Monee, IL
20 November 2024

70664043R00079